basic facts of
BODY WATER AND IONS

basic facts
of
BODY WATER
AND IONS

SECOND EDITION

By STEWART M. BROOKS, M.S.

Formerly Instructor in Science and Pharmacology, Lasell Junior College, Auburndale, Massachusetts, and Boston City Hospital School of Nursing, Boston, Massachusetts

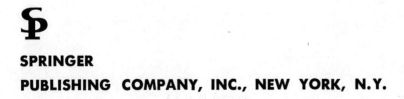

SPRINGER
PUBLISHING COMPANY, INC., NEW YORK, N.Y.

AND ONCE AGAIN

TO

NAT AND MARSHALL

PREFACE TO THE SECOND EDITION

This book has been written for those who seek a basic understanding of the body's fluid and electrolyte balance in health and disease. Even though eight years have passed since the publication of the first edition, this work continues to be the only one of its kind that is especially addressed to nurses. The absence of competition, however, has in no way led to complacency on the part of the author; quite to the contrary. The writing of the present edition proved more difficult because of numerous suggestions, reappraisals, expanded knowledge, and the desire to make the text at once clear, concise, accurate, and complete. The second edition represents new flesh on what is apparently a tried and true skeleton. Hopefully, the book will continue to serve as a standard work in clinical medicine for the nurse, and as a quick refresher of the basic facts for the doctor and intern.

The author wishes to express his deep appreciation to Abbott Laboratories of North Chicago, Illinois; Baxter Laboratories, Morton Grove, Illinois; and Cutter Laboratories of Berkeley, California, for their generous permission to use and modify illustrative material. The author wishes to thank once again Mrs. Marie E. Litterer for providing the excellent artwork. Finally, the author thanks his wonderful wife for sharing in the backbreaking but glorious experience of writing a book.

STEWART M. BROOKS

Auburndale, Massachusetts
December, 1967

CONTENTS

Solutions:

PART ONE

THE FACTS EXPLAINED

I

INTRODUCTION

The great bulk of living matter is just plain water, yet historically speaking, the subject of water and electrolyte balance is a newcomer to the art and science of bedside medicine. This is not to imply, of course, that our grandparents did not know enough to take a drink of water to quench their thirst. Indeed they did—but often to their detriment! Drinking plain water in response to excessive sweating, for example, results in "heat cramps" unless salt is also taken. Today this is common knowledge—sweat contains salt as well as water—but years ago this relationship was either unknown or not appreciated.

It was just about fifty years ago that the patient in the hospital began to receive the benefits of both salt and water in the treatment and prophylaxis of dehydration, but eventually the shortcomings of plain salt and water were disclosed and the complexities of body fluid disturbances brought to light. Protracted diarrhea, for instance, can be fatal despite the replacement of salt and water unless the doctor also administers potassium and bicarbonate. Conversely, the administration of potassium to a patient with acute renal disease can cause immediate death . . . And so on.

In sum, then, the subject of body fluids—that is, water and electrolytes—is of life and death importance and it behooves the nurse to both understand and appreciate the principles of the subject as they apply to the bedside situation. This is a fascinating study which, at the elementary level, yields to a pinch of science and a handful of common sense.

Our approach will be as follows: First, to understand completely the basic facts of body water, body ions, and body pH in health and disease and then to apply this knowledge to the basic treatment of specific diseases (see Fig. 1). Although, as indicated, water, ions and pH can rarely be divorced from one another at the bedside, for obvious pedagogic reasons they are best discussed in separate chapters. And so let us now begin.

3

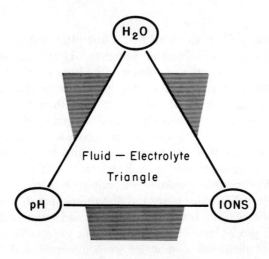

Figure 1: The basic elements of the body's fluid and electrolyte system.

II

WATER

The total body water of the adult male ranges between 50 and 70 percent of his total body weight; that of the adult female from 44 to 65 percent. Water content clearly varies with each individual and is related mainly to the fat content of the body; relatively little water is associated with fat. Since the female has a significantly greater amount of body fat than has the male, we can easily appreciate the aforementioned percentages. In obese people (35 percent fat) the water content may drop to as low as 43 percent of the total body weight compared to thin people (8 percent fat) with a water content of 70 percent. This is of much more than academic interest because the obese patient is certainly not going to do as well with a dehydrating illness.

Then there is the matter of age. The newborn infant has a water content of 70 to 83 percent of its total body weight! At six months, this figure has dropped precipitously to about 60 percent, followed by a very slow decline to somewhere around 55 percent at ten years of age or thereabouts. At this time the male commences on a path of "rehydration," reaching a peak of 70 percent at about the age of twenty-five, followed once again by a gradual decline to 60 percent at the age of fifty—a figure which holds pretty steady for the remaining years of life. In contrast, the female merely continues to lose more water over her growing years, and attains a steady figure of 45 percent or so at the age of fifty. These percentages may be of considerable concern during illness associated with dehydration, particularly dehydration in the infant. During the first year of life fluid derangements are commonly serious.

5

The compartments

For clinical purposes, the authorities tell us that we may take a middle-of-the-road figure of 60 percent as the total water content of the body; that is, 60 percent of the total body weight (Fig. 2). By way of example, a 70 kilogram individual would contain in his body 42 kilograms of water or, in more familiar terms, 42 liters. (One kilogram of water occupies a volume of one liter.) Further, of this volume of 42 liters we may consider 28 liters (40 percent of the total body weight) as the water present within the cells (intracellular compartment) and 14 liters (20 percent of the total body weight) as water present outside the cells (extracellular compartment). Finally, of this extracellular volume 10.5 liters (15 percent of the total body weight) surround the cells proper (intercellular or interstitial compartment) and 3.5 liters (5 percent) are confined to the blood (plasma compartment). Note especially that 60 percent (total body water) equals 40 percent (intracellular water) plus 15 percent (intercellular water) plus 5 percent (plasma water).

Let us take another example. Suppose the person weighs 60 kilograms. Here the total body water is 60 percent of 60, or 36 liters; the intracellular water is 40 percent of 60, or 24 liters; the extracellular water is 20 percent of 60, or 12 liters, of which 9 liters is interstitial (15 percent of 60) and 3 liters (5 percent of 60) plasma water. As a way of a check, we note that 24 liters plus 9 liters plus 3 liters equals 36 liters.

Balance and osmosis

Our next concern is the miraculous way in which the body is able to maintain—or *balance*—the compartments at their respective volumes (see Fig. 3).

The boundary between the intracellular and intercellular compartments is obviously the sum total of all the cellular membranes, and central to the idea of compartmental water balance is the fact that the cellular membrane is, among myriad other things, semipermeable; that is, it easily permits the free movement of water molecules, but partially or completely prevents

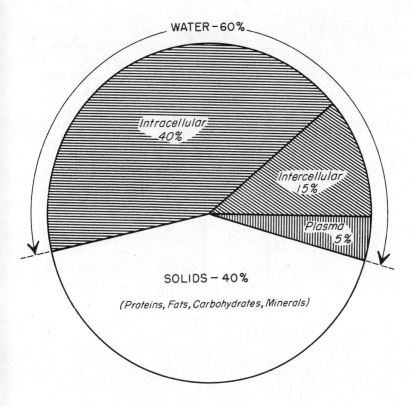

Figure 2: Composition of body and distribution of its water.

The overall balance

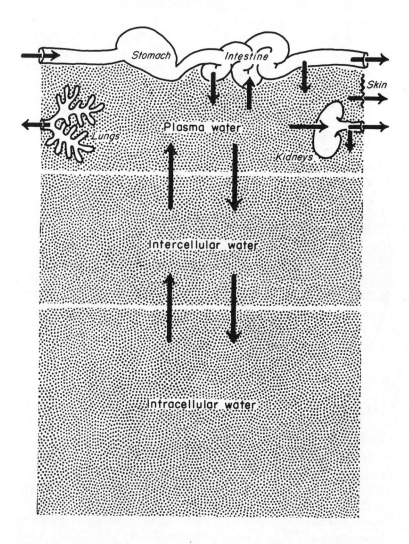

Figure 3: Distribution and movement of body water (modified from Gamble).

the passage of other particles. When such a membrane separates two aqueous solutions with different densities, the principal flow of water across the membrane will be in the direction of the solution with the greater density. (By *density,* or *osmotic density,* we mean the proportion of particles—ions and molecules—to volume). This will continue until the two solutions are of the same density, at which time the rate of flow will be the same in both directions. The flow of water across a semipermeable membrane as a consequence of a difference in density is called *osmosis,* and the rule is, as just stated, that the principal flow will be from the less dense to the more dense. There is one way to always remember this and that is by common sense: the least dense solution has the most water.

In health, the concentrations of the intercellular and intracellular compartments are such that at osmotic equilibrium the water distribution is 15 percent and 40 percent, respectively. When these concentrations are disturbed we can easily understand the consequences. For example, a drop in the concentration of salt (the chief solute) in the intercellular compartment would cause abnormal amounts of water to flow into the cells; conversely, an increase in the concentration of salt in that compartment would remove water from the cells.

Shifting our attention a little, we note that the intercellular compartment borders the plasma compartment as well as the intracellular compartment, thereby effecting a second osmotic system—this time with the capillary wall serving as the semipermeable membrane. Here water is forced out of the capillaries by the hydrostatic pressure of the blood and pulled into the capillaries by the osmotic (or oncotic) pull of plasma protein (Fig. 4). Essentially, then, the maintenance—and balance—of the water content of the plasma (5 percent) and intercellular (15 percent) compartments depends upon the blood pressure and plasma protein concentration. In malnutrition, for instance, there is a drop in plasma protein with the result that excessive amounts of water are lost to the intercellular compartment, causing edema and swollen bellies. Conversely, in dehydration, the loss of water from the plasma causes a relative increase in pro-

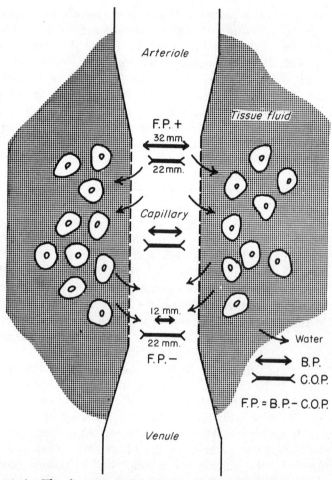

Figure 4: The formation of tissue, or interstitial, fluid. At the arteriolar end of capillary, fluid is forced out through the capillary wall because the blood's hydrostatic pressure (B.P.) exceeds the blood's colloidal osmotic pressure (C.O.P.); i.e., the so-called filtration pressure (F.P.) is about 10 mm. (32 mm. — 22 mm.). At the venular end, however, the situation is reversed because the B.P. drops while the C.O.P. remains the same; i.e., fluid is "drawn" into the capillary by a pressure of about 10 mm. (22 — 12). Thus, the overall effect is "balance."

tein concentration with the result that water, this time, is "lost" to the capillaries.

Let us now integrate our knowledge of compartmental balance by considering an actual derangement. The drinking of amounts of water over and above what the body needs can cause a serious, acute condition aptly called water intoxication, and this is what happens: Water taken into the body is absorbed into the blood—the plasma compartment—thus increasing blood volume and, thereby, blood pressure. As a result of this increased pressure, water is forced through the capillary walls into the intercellular compartment. The intercellular compartment now becomes more dilute, meaning that water will leave it and pass into the now relatively more concentrated intracellular compartment. Thus, the underlying pathology of water intoxication is excessive cellular hydration. But of chief interest to us at this point is that an alteration in one compartment is reflected by alterations in the other two. One further example should crystallize this fact.

When one drinks excessive amounts of salt water, the kidney is not able to prevent a build-up of salt in the intercellular compartment, with the result that water will be withdrawn from the intracellular compartment into the intercellular and plasma compartments, in that order. This means, of course, that the blood pressure will increase (as a result of an increase in blood volume) and the output of urine will be increased. Indeed, for each quart of sea water the castaway drinks, he eliminates a quart and a half of urine, with the difference coming from the cells. Cause of death—dehydration; lesson for the student—an alteration in one compartment causes alterations in the other two.

Alimentary balance

A rather special form of compartmental balance is the relationship between plasma water and alimentary secretions—the latter being derived from the former. According to J. L. Gamble, the total volume of alimentary secretions during a twenty-four-hour period may reach the staggering volume of 8200 ml. or 8.2 liters (Fig. 5) and, what is more, all but about 150 ml. or so is

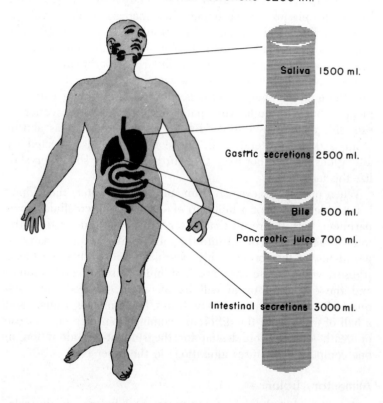

Figure 5: Digestive secretions in adult. (Redrawn from *Fluid and Electrolytes*, 1960. Courtesy of Abbott Laboratories, North Chicago, Illinois.)

returned to the circulation incident to reabsorption in the intestine (Fig. 4). No wonder, then, that protracted vomiting or diarrhea—without fluid replacement—can cause death in a matter of hours. About this much more will be said, for fluid derangements in the wake of such alimentary losses (and the treatment thereof) epitomize the entire subject of body water and ions.

Water intake vs. water output

Living organisms vary tremendously in their water requirements. Whereas a cactus can live for twenty-nine years on an amount of water equal to its own weight, it takes man only a month to drink his weight in water. But regardless of the quantity imbibed, the body normally balances the gain with an equivalent loss, or, put another way, the body takes in an amount of water equal to that which it loses. The important thing is to maintain balance, and the body is outstandingly successful in this regard. At twenty-four-hour intervals man's weight may vary less than one-half pound! The regulating mechanisms involved will be discussed later.

Intake

In a typical day, a man may gain close to 3 liters of water. This includes not only imbibed water, but also the water that is trapped in food or derived from oxidation of food (Fig. 6). Imbibed water heads the list with a volume of about 1.5 liters per day. The water in food, so-called preformed water, contributes about half this amount. Foods contain a surprisingly large quantity of water. Green vegetables, for example, are around 95 percent water; and meat, 50 to 75 percent. Oxidative water refers to the water formed as a by-product in the body's oxidation of foods; this amounts to about one-half the volume of preformed water. Roughly, these three volumes present an easily-remembered ratio of 4-2-1 (imbibed, preformed, and oxidative).

Thus, the food intake has a great bearing on the body's need for imbibed fluid. In anuria, where every drop of water must be reckoned with, preformed water and oxidative water must be considered with the same seriousness as the water tap. The

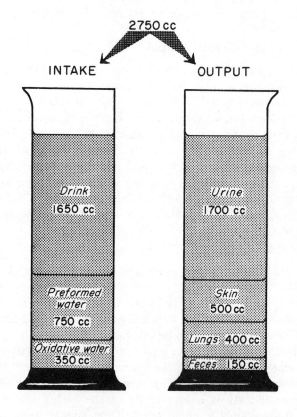

Figure 6: Water intake vs. output in a typical day. (Modified, from Wolf, A. V., Body water. *Scientific American,* November, 1958.)

kangaroo rat of the desert illustrates these facts; it never takes a drink as long as it lives, deriving its water solely from food! If man lived on cucumbers, he would be equally distinguished.

Imbibed water is rapidly absorbed into the plasma compartment; in the absence of food the process takes less than an hour. The immediate effect is an increase in blood volume and blood pressure, which in turn opens up "inactive" capillary networks and the sinusoids of the liver and spleen. As a result, there is a shift of water to the intercellular compartment. Finally, since an increase in intercellular water lowers the osmotic pressure of that compartment, there is now a shift of water to the intracellular areas.

The role the kidneys play during this adjustment period will depend upon the body's water status prior to imbibition. If there is hemoconcentration (as a result of a water deficit) the kidney will allow the compartments to attain their normal volume before removing any water from the blood. Excess water, of course, is readily eliminated.

Output

Now let us take a look at the body's water output (Fig. 6). To balance the intake, the output runs close to 3 liters in a typical day. As one would guess, the kidneys carry the heaviest load (e.g., 1.7 liters). The other channels of excretion are not as apparent, but are nonetheless vital. Under usual conditions, the body loses about 0.5 liter from the skin and 0.4 liter from the lungs. The remainder, 0.2 liter or so, is lost in the feces.

In contrast to fecal water and urine, the water lost via the lungs is in the form of vapor. Water lost through the skin is usually vapor, but can turn into water (sweat) when the body becomes overheated. We employ the term "insensible perspiration" when referring to invisible sweat, or water vapor.

The kidney

One of the functions of the kidney is to maintain water and electrolyte balance. For this reason we must pay special attention to it and to its relationship to other forces in the body. For the present, we shall confine our discussion to the handling of water.

The unit of the kidney is the nephron (Fig. 7), of which there are about one million in each organ. To call it a microscopic filtering device is permissible so long as we understand *how* it filters.

The caliber of the afferent vessel leading to the tuft of capillaries, or glomerulus, is appreciably larger than that of the efferent vessel. This results in a substantial filtration pressure which causes water to be forced through the capillary wall. This so-called glomerular filtrate represents an aqueous solution of the blood's water-soluble constituents—urea, salt, glucose, and so on; it contains no blood cells and almost no protein. The filtrate is "caught" in Bowman's capsule and then starts on its tortuous sojourn through the tubules. By the time it reaches the *collecting* tubule (which empties into the pelvis of the kidney) it is urine.

What happens is simple enough in principle. The tubule walls reabsorb water and the so-called threshold constituents—glucose, ions, and the like—back into the blood. Reabsorption, however, takes place only to the extent of keeping the internal environment on an even keel, i.e., to maintain homeostasis. In states of dehydration, for example, practically all water is re-absorbed. On the other hand, when the body has an excess of water, less will be reabsorbed. In the former case, then, the volume of urine will be much less than in the latter, and its specific gravity will be higher.

The same principle holds for threshold substances. In diabetes, for example, the tubule walls will not reabsorb all the glucose from the filtrate, for the blood has too much already. Consequently, sugar will appear in the urine (glycosuria). Wastes, or nonthreshold substances such as urea, are not actively reab-sorbed. Thus, urine is an aqueous solution of "unwanted chemicals." Although each nephron manufactures only a fraction of a drop, two million nephrons, taken together, can produce considerable amounts of urine.

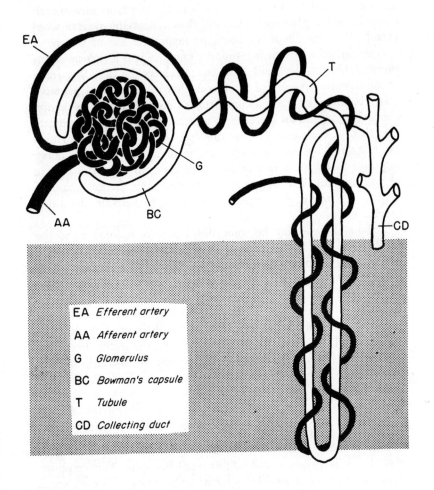

Figure 7: The nephron (see text for explanation of function).

EA *Efferent artery*

AA *Afferent artery*

G *Glomerulus*

BC *Bowman's capsule*

T *Tubule*

CD *Collecting duct*

Vasopressin

The kidney is definitely subject to outside influences. One is the hormone vasopressin, or antidiuretic hormone (ADH), of the posterior pituitary. In some subtle biochemical fashion, this hormone stimulates the tubule walls of the nephron to reabsorb water from the glomerular filtrate, thus conserving water. Conversely, the absence of the hormone favors the loss of water.

How does the posterior pituitary "know" when to release vasopressin? One widely held explanation relates the initiating force to the osmotic pressure of the blood; that is, in states of negative water balance the plasma compartment contracts, causing hemoconcentration and an increase in osmotic pressure. According to this theory, certain cells (osmoreceptors) in the hypothalamus are triggered by the elevated osmotic pressure to release nerve impulses to the posterior pituitary, causing, in turn, the release of vasopressin. The opposite occurs following the ingestion of water. (Osmoreceptors are also believed to activate the thirst mechanisms.)

Although there may be some differences of opinion as to the mechanism that triggers the release of vasopressin, no one will dispute the hormone's pronounced action on the kidney. This action is well illustrated by the disease known as diabetes insipidus. The characteristic sign here is the elimination of huge volumes of urine. Also, of course, large volumes of water are ingested to maintain balance. What has happened is that the tubule wall has lost its ability to reabsorb water from the glomerular filtrate, the cause being a lack of vasopressin. Administration of the hormone readily restores the body to a normal water balance.

Circulation

Since the production of the glomerular filtrate depends upon a certain pressure within the glomerulus, it stands to reason that a drop in blood pressure will inhibit renal function. This response, however, may be desirable as far as water balance is concerned. In hemorrhage, for instance, the drop in blood volume means a drop in blood pressure and a lessened flow of urine. Water is thus retained in an attempt to prevent a negative balance.

Diuretics

Diuretics are agents that stimulate the production of urine. The chief natural diuretic, of course, is water. Following the intake of water the plasma compartment increases in volume, causing a temporary rise in blood pressure and a lowering of osmotic pressure. The former response favors the manufacture of the glomerular filtrate, and the latter a decreased output of vasopressin (meaning less tubular reabsorption of water). Consequently, there is a substantial increase in urine output.

Actually, an infinite number of substances, in addition to water, have a diuretic action. Urea, for example, is another natural diuretic. Being a nonthreshold substance it is forced to remain in the tubule and, in so doing, holds water. This means more urine. Theoretically, any nonthreshold substance is a diuretic. The diuretics employed as drugs are much more potent and operate through a different mechanism. Essentially, they act by inhibiting the tubular reabsorption of Na^+ and Cl^-. Forced to remain in the tubule, these ions hold water which the tubule wall is temporarily unable to reabsorb back into the blood. As a result, there is a tremendous outpouring of urine; in edematous conditions, a single injection effects the removal of 10 to 20 liters of water.

The skin and the lungs

Whereas the kidney in health always operates to maintain water balance, the same cannot be said of the skin. The loss of water through the skin serves not only to remove wastes, but also to maintain body temperature. In the tropics, for example, while the kidney fights dehydration by putting out a low volume of urine, the skin fights the heat by allowing 10 to 12 liters of water to evaporate per day.

The sweat, or sudoriferous, glands lie deep in the true skin and their secretions—perspiration—are carried to the surface by corkscrew-like ducts. The work of these glands is governed by sympathetic nerves which, in turn, are under the direction of a hypothetical "sweat center" in the brain (perhaps in the hypothalamus). As the temperature of the blood rises, chiefly in response to the external temperature and/or muscular activity, the heat center is triggered to send impulses via sympathetic fibers to the glands. Sweat is thus formed and the body is cooled by evaporation. The sweat seen in many emotional conditions—the "cold sweat" of fear, for example—is easily explained by the emergency nature of the sympathetic system.

Perspiration, about 99 percent water, contains dissolved salts (chiefly NaCl) and traces of urea. In abnormal conditions, however, bile pigments, albumin, sugar or even blood may appear in perspiration. The output on a typical day ranges around 0.5 liter.

The water lost by the lungs averages about 0.4 liter per day. Since this is a case of simple evaporation, the loss is constant and largely unaffected by other factors.

III

IONS

Whereas plain water does not conduct an electric current, the fluids of the body do conduct a current, demonstrating quite clearly that such fluids are actually aqueous solutions of electrolytes. As we know, electrolytes dissociate into charged particles called ions, and in the instance of the body those of principal concern are the cations (positive ions) sodium (Na^+), potassium (K^+), calcium (Ca^{++}), and magnesium (Mg^{++}) and the anions (negative ions) chloride (Cl^-), bicarbonate (HCO_3^-), and phosphate ($HPO_4^=$).

The milliequivalent

Chemically and physiologically the best way to express ionic concentration is in terms of milliequivalents per liter (mEq./L.), a milliequivalent being the amount (Fig. 8) of one ion that will exactly react with or replace a milliequivalent of any other ion. For example, one milliequivalent of Na^+ will exactly react with one milliequivalent of Cl^-; two milliequivalents of Na^+ will exactly react with two milliequivalents of Cl^-; and so on. Further, a solution of any electrolyte of any concentration contains the same number of milliequivalents of anion and cation. For example, normal saline solution (0.9 percent sodium chloride) contains 154 milliequivalents of Na^+ and 154 milliequivalents of Cl^- per liter. And, of course, this applies to "multiple electrolyte"; that is, if we were to add a pinch of $NaHCO_3$, a pinch of K_2SO_4 and a pinch of $CaCl_2$ to a beaker of distilled water, the total milliequivalents of cation (Na^+, K^+ and Ca^{++}) would equal the total milliequivalents of anion (HCO_3^-, $SO_4^=$, Cl^-).

21

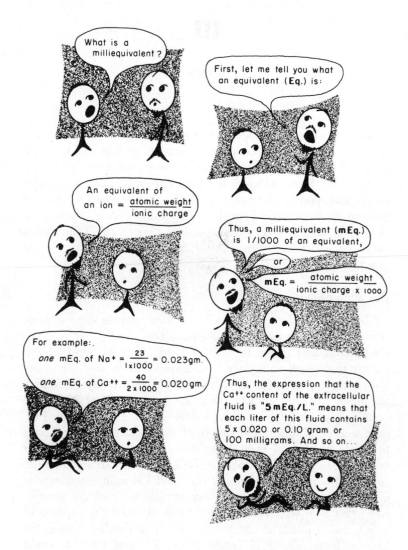

Figure 8: An "ionic conversation" worth listening to.

Extracellular electrolytes

The essential chemical difference between the plasma and intercellular compartments relates solely to protein, with concentrations of 16 mEq./L. and 1 mEq./L. per liter, respectively. (For body electrolyte purposes proteins are considered to be anions.) Otherwise the ionic patterns of the two compartments are so close that they are generally considered to be one in most clinical situations relating to electrolyte balance. As vividly depicted in Fig. 9, the chief cation is, by far, Na^+, with an average concentration of 142 mEq./L. The concentration of K^+ and Ca^{++} may each be taken as 5 mEq./L., and that of Mg^{++} as 3 mEq./L. Hardly as a surprise, Cl^-, with a concentration of 103 mEq./L., is the chief anion. The average concentrations of HCO_3^- and $HPO_4^=$ are 27 and 2, respectively. The total concentration of cation and total concentration of anion hover, in health, close to the value of 155 mEq/L.

Intracellular electrolytes

A comparison of Figures 9 and 10 shows the considerable difference between the extracellular and intracellular fluid compartments, a difference which the physiologist and biochemist have still not been able to explain to everyone's satisfaction. Obviously, sodium and potassium pass across the cellular membrane (not as freely as water, of course). How then do we explain the cell's retention of potassium (125 mEq./L.) and rejection of sodium (10 mEq./L.) and chloride (5 mEq./L.)? It certainly has nothing to do with particle size because K^+ is actually larger than Na^+. A recent view is that the cell membrane does indeed permit the entrance of sodium into the cell, meaning that some sort of metabolic pump is in continuous operation to return the ion back across the membrane into the interstitial fluid. In other words, the difference in concentration is a consequence of an active process which the cell maintains according to the metabolic dictates of nature—a demand for much more K^+ than Na^+.

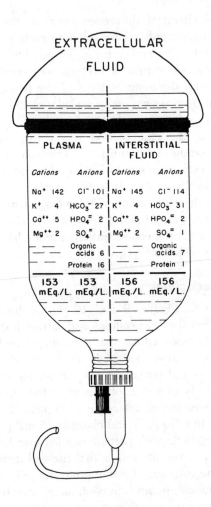

Figure 9: Note that the only major difference between the plasma and interstitial fluid relates to the content of protein. Ionically, they are just about the same and invariably considered as such.

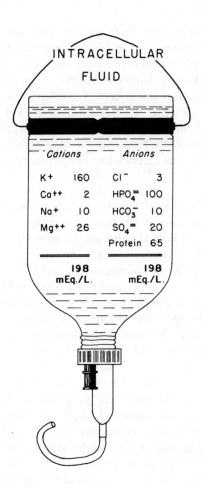

Figure 10: The ionic profile of the intracellular fluid. Note that total milliequivalents (mEq.) of cation (positive ions) always equal total milliequivalents of anion (negative ions).

Balance

The electroyle balance between the intracellular and extracellular compartments is, as indicated, predicated upon the functional integrity of the cellular membrane. Too, there is, as with water, an "alimentary balance," for the 6 to 8 liters of fluid—containing prodigious amounts of electrolyte—released to the alimentary tract during a twenty-four-hour period are ultimately reabsorbed back into the blood and distributed about the extracellular compartment. Thus, the damage resulting from vomiting and diarrhea arises from a loss of electrolyte as well as water.

The kidney

Electrolyte balance at the compartmental level is plainly and inextricably associated with the intake-output regulation—a responsibility which falls almost entirely upon the kidney. Indeed, for all practical purposes, the total sodium excreted in the urine per 24 hours equals the sodium intake and varies with diet. The average range for sodium chloride excretion is between 3 and 8 grams daily. Interestingly, the sodium output bears a somewhat inverse relationship to the output of potassium (which averages 3.5 grams per day) because of the action of the adrenal cortical hormone aldosterone. This is to say, the hormone stimulates the kidney tubule to reabsorb sodium and reject potassium. With the reabsorption of sodium there is also a concomitant reabsorption of water since the ion is always hydrated. The adrenals step up their output of aldosterone in such stressful situations as extreme dehydration and hemorrhage, thereby conserving sodium and water and aiding in the maintenance of blood volume—and blood pressure. The chief mechanism for the conservation of water, however, relates to the action of the anti-diuretic hormone, vasopressin.

The skin

Under normal conditions and in temperate climates electrolyte loss from the skin is negligible (from 0.4 to 0.8 gram daily) but with increased environmental temperature, fever or muscular exercise the loss of sodium may become marked. The concentration of sodium in sweat is usually about 27 mEq./L., though it may be as high as 100 mEq./L. Loss of sodium in sweat is a by-product of temperature regulation. Under abnormal conditions such loss may be undesirable from the viewpoint of electrolyte balance, yet obligatory to maintain normal temperature. Indeed, a total day's intake of sodium may be dissipated in the sweat in 6 to 8 hours under adverse conditions.

Alimentary tract

Though the alimentary tract is the usual pathological avenue of fluid and electrolyte loss, under normal conditions the output here is less than from the skin. The normal daily loss of sodium chloride in the feces ranges somewhere around 0.2 gram.

IV

pH

The topic of body fluids is, as we know, a "triangular affair" two sides of which—water and electrolytes (ions)—we have already discussed. The third side is pH, which is an arithmetic expression of a solution's acidity or alkalinity. Specifically, a solution with a pH of 7 is neutral; that is, it contains an equal number of hydrogen ions and hydroxyl ions. A solution with a pH below 7 is acid; that is, it contains more hydrogen ions that hydroxyl ions. A solution with a pH above 7 is alkaline (or basic); that is, it contains more hydroxyl ions than hydrogen ions. The so-called pH scale runs from 0 to 14, with "pure" acid (0) and "pure" base (14) to the left and right of neutrality (7), respectively. Of special interest to us in our work is that pH is a means of expressing the exact degree of acidity or alkalinity. For instance, a solution with a pH of 7.4 is just slightly less basic than a solution with a pH of 7.5, and so on.

Buffers

Having said this let us turn to the interesting physiological fact that if the pH of the extracellular compartment (i.e., the plasma and interstitial fluid) strays just slightly from the range of 7.35 to 7.45 the body is in for trouble (Fig. 11). Below 7.35 the result is acidosis, and above it alkalosis; below 6.8 or above 8 the result is death! Considering the galaxy of acidic and basic materials entering the blood from without and within, and considering that only a drop of acid or base can swing the pH of a gallon of water a noticeable distance from center, we begin to appreciate the re-

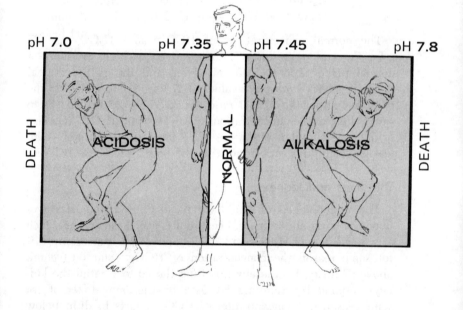

pH 7.0   pH 7.35   pH 7.45   pH 7.8

DEATH   ACIDOSIS   NORMAL   ALKALOSIS   DEATH

Figure 11: The life-and-death role of pH. (From *Parenteral Solutions Handbook*, 1965. Courtesy of Cutter Laboratories, Berkeley, California).

markable machinery the body has developed to keep the pH where it belongs—or in balance.

Actually the complexities of this system, even to the senior chemistry student, can be formidable, but it deserves to be stressed over and over again that, for all intents and purposes, at the bedside the matter is quite simple.

In essence, the extracellular compartment is immunized against pH changes by the presence of so-called buffer systems, the most important of which is bicarbonate-carbonic acid ($[HCO_3^-]$-$[H_2CO_3]$). Carbonic acid, as we know from chemistry, neutralizes bases, and bicarbonate converts strong acids to the weak acid H_2CO_3. Thus:

$$H_2CO_3 + OH^- \longrightarrow HCO_3^- + H_2O$$
$$HCO_3^- + H^+ \longrightarrow H_2CO_3$$

The normal concentrations of HCO_3^- and H_2CO_3 are 27 mEq./L. and 1.33 mEq./L., respectively, which produces a normal pH of 7.35 to 7.45. However—and this is the critical point—it is not the *absolute* values of 27 versus 1.33 which do the trick, but rather the 20 to 1 *ratio* (i.e., 27:1.33::20:1). That is to say, as long as the concentrations of HCO_3^- and H_2CO_3 increase or decrease simultaneously, the pH is maintained. In more clinical language, this ratio represents the body's acid-base balance.

The lungs and kidneys

The maintenance of acid-base balance ultimately devolves upon the lungs and kidneys, because it is just these organs which are the arbiters of H_2CO_3 and HCO_3^- (Fig. 12). For example, if for some reason the concentration of HCO_3^- starts to climb above 27 mEq./L.—thereby upsetting the 20 to 1 ratio—the kidneys respond by excreting HCO_3^-; by the same token if for some reason the concentration of HCO_3^- starts to drop below 27—thereby again upsetting the 20 to 1 ratio—the kidneys conserve HCO_3^-. And, in conjunction with this mechanism, the kidneys excrete or conserve hydrogen ions (acid) according to the desired effect. For example, if the pH of the blood starts to

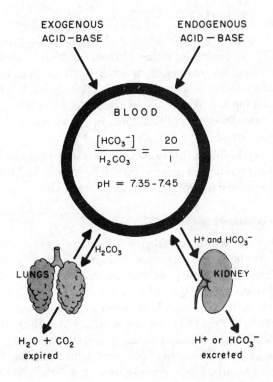

Figure 12: The regulation of blood pH. As long as the lungs and kidneys maintain a 20-to-1 ratio of the bicarbonate-carbonic acid buffer system, the pH will remain 7.35-7.45 even though acidic and basic substances are continuously entering the bloodstream from without (exogenous) and from within (endogenous).

move its way up, the kidneys respond by conserving hydrogen ions (acid); conversely, if the pH starts to drop, the kidneys excrete hydrogen ions.

An analogous mechanism prevails in the lung. The carbon dioxide we exhale comes from carbonic acid, that is,

$$H_2CO_3 \longrightarrow H_2O + CO_2$$

The meaning here is clear because the more CO_2 exhaled the more H_2CO_3 is, obviously, removed from the blood. Thus, if the pH of the blood for one reason or other starts to drop, there is a compensatory increase in respiration. (Hold your breath for a firsthand example!) Again, an increase in pH is met with decreased respiration. (Hyperventilate for a minute or so for a firsthand example.)

To repeat, the lungs, by exhaling or conserving CO_2, and the kidneys, by excreting or conserving HCO_3^- and hydrogen ions, are constantly striving to maintain acid-base balance.

Acidosis–alkalosis

An upset in acid-base balance results in either acidosis or alkalosis. If there is an increase in blood carbonic acid or decrease in blood bicarbonate (thereby decreasing the 20 to 1 ratio) the result is acidosis. Conversely, if there is an increase in blood bicarbonate or decrease in blood carbonic acid (thereby increasing the 20 to 1 ratio) the upshot is alkalosis. Thus, there are two kinds of alkalosis and acidosis: respiratory (arising from an alteration of carbonic acid) and metabolic (arising from an alteration in bicarbonate). For instance, metabolic alkalosis is an acid-base imbalance caused by an increase in bicarbonate. Equally significant, a given imbalance is either compensated or uncompensated, depending upon whether the lungs and kidneys, in the manner just described, are able to restore the altered ratio and thereby maintain the pH. If it is maintained the situation is said to be compensated; otherwise it is uncompensated. For example, in compensated metabolic acidosis the pH is maintained even though there is a decrease in blood bicarbonate.

V

IMBALANCES

In disturbances of body fluids there is an imbalance of water, electrolytes and/or pH; the most common situations—vomiting and diarrhea—involve a loss of *both* water and electrolytes. In extreme cases all three factors are often askew. For instance, whereas in mild vomiting and diarrhea the imbalances relate to lost water and electrolytes, in protracted cases the pH also changes; that is, an excessive loss of acid (HCl) incident to vomiting incites an alkalosis, and an excessive loss of base (HCO_3^-) incident to diarrhea incites acidosis. Other conditions underscored by disturbances of body fluids include hemorrhage, burns, heat exhaustion, polyuria, edema, diabetes mellitus and acute kidney failure.

In addition, we must be ever mindful of the relationship certain drugs bear to body water, electrolytes and acid-base balance. Some incite an imbalance (e.g., ACTH, corticosteroids, diuretics and sodium bicarbonate), while others effect unusual pharmacological responses in the face of a pre-existing imbalance. For instance, potassium antagonizes the action of digitalis, which means that an otherwise harmless dose of that drug may evoke intoxication in the face of hypokalemia. This is especially noteworthy because heart patients are often treated with both digitalis and diuretics; the latter commonly cause hypokalemia unless supplemental potassium (e.g., KCl) is administered prophylactically. Again, the intravenous administration of a calcium salt can result in sudden death in the digitalized patient. Thus, 1) be on the alert for drugs which could possibly incite an imbalance; 2) make sure the patient is "in balance" before administering potent drugs; 3) always consider the interplay of electrolyte and drug when their concomitant administration is contemplated.

States of imbalance

In most instances a given fluid and electrolyte disturbance can be characterized by one or *more* of the following expressions: dehydration (loss of fluid), edema (excess fluid), hyponatremia (excess sodium), hypokalemia (loss of potassium), hyperkalemia (excess potassium), acidosis (decrease in pH) and alkalosis (increase in pH). For example, severe diarrhea can result in dehydration, hyponatremia, hypokalemia and acidosis. All of which means, of course, that severe diarrhea produces a clinical picture whose signs and symptoms arise from an interplay of at least four factors—a loss of sodium, a loss of potassium, a loss of water and a decreased pH. Thus fluid and electrolyte disturbances are characteristically "multiple situations." Nonetheless, we shall find it worth while to consider each of the aforesaid states (dehydration, etc.) individually because it is indeed true that such states, rare though they are, can exist alone. For example, the seriously ill patient who is being maintained solely by vein might well die if the fluids used did not contain potassium. Cause of death: hypokalemia.

Dehydration

The clinical state which follows in the wake of the abnormal loss of fluid—dehydration—is one of the first problems that comes to mind in a discussion of body fluids. Dehydration also occurs when a normal loss is not offset by a normal intake. Actually, dehydration is somewhat of a misnomer because the body rarely loses *just* water. The real loss is fluid; that is, water plus electrolytes, and the classical signs and symptoms (of dehydration) relate to both factors. The familiar signs include loss of turgor of the skin, sunken eyes, dryness of the mucous membranes, and loss of body weight, the latter being the best index of the condition. When the loss of water predominates over that of electrolyte, thirst is particularly prominent although, to a lesser extent, a fall in volume alone may incite a desire for water. In severe cases the aforesaid picture represents the prelude to the full-blown symptoms of weakness, anorexia, nausea and vomiting, renal failure, shock and, ultimately, coma.

Edema

Diametrically opposed to dehydration is edema, or the presence of abnormally large amounts of fluid in the interstitial compartment. The causes are many—capillary damage, failing heart, hypoproteinemia and obstructed lymphatics, to name the most significant. Unfortunately, edema is a self-perpetuating condition; that is, as a result of the loss of fluid from the plasma compartment to the interstitial compartment there is a drop in blood volume which brings about the release of aldosterone and ADH and the conservation of electrolytes and water, respectively. Actually this would be physiologically sensible if it were not for the fact that the fluid so retained is promptly lost to the interstitial compartment, thereby worsening an already serious situation.

Sodium

A deficit of sodium (hyponatremia) may result from lack of sodium intake, extreme losses through perspiration, excessive gastrointestinal discharge, or inordinate losses in the urine stemming from an adrenal insufficiency. Hyponatremia is rapidly reflected in the absence of both sodium and chloride in the urine. The effects of hyponatremia are poor renal blood flow, altered water balance, dehydration, dizziness, nausea, hypotension and, in extreme cases, stupor and convulsions. The opposite situation, or hypernatremia, (or excess sodium), generally stems from over-administration of sodium chloride. Too, hypernatremia may occur incident to congestive heart failure and the use of such drugs as deoxycorticosterone. Because the sodium ion has an affinity for water the cardinal sign is edema.

Chloride

Chloride, the chief anion of the extracellular compartment, has close ties with sodium: both ions are generally ingested together (as NaCl), reabsorbed together (by the kidney) and, in the face of impaired renal function, may be lost together. However, chloride is most rapidly excreted as KCl and in most cases of a potassium deficiency (hypokalemia) there is a concomitant chloride deficiency (hypochloremia). The signs and symptoms of hypochloremia are inextricably related to those associated with hypokalemia and hyponatremia.

Potassium

Potassium is the chief cation of the intracellular compartment; the total amount in a 70 kg. man is in the neighborhood of 4000 mEq.—two-thirds of which is bound to protein. Because the unbound third can, under certain conditions, pass across the cell wall and cause an obligatory influx of H^+ ions into the cell (to balance the loss) we see that potassium has a decided bearing on acid-base balance.

Hypokalemia (or hypopotassemia) develops rapidly unless an adequate intake of potassium is maintained. Also, the state arises in any case where there is an abnormal cell breakdown; that is, the protein-bound ion becomes unleashed and passes into the extracellular compartment, whereupon the renal tubules place it into the urine. Other causes of hypokalemia include stress, vomiting, diarrhea, fistulae, gastric and intestinal suction, diabetic acidosis, and excessive administration of potassium-free fluids, sodium, ACTH, and adrenal cortical hormones.

The clinical symptoms of hypokalemia are weakness in the extremities, flaccid paralysis, muscular twitchings, weakness and paralysis of the respiratory muscles, an irregular pulse and, in the post-operative patient, abdominal distention. Highly characteristic, too, are changes in the electrocardiogram (Fig. 13). Finally, most instances of hypokalemia are accompanied by and associated with hypochloremia and alkalosis.

Also a threat to life is hyperkalemia, which is usually a consequence of excessive administration of the ion in patients unable to excrete it or a result of the release of excessive potassium from the intracellular compartment incident to cellular destruction. In acute kidney failure hyperkalemia is now believed to be the chief culprit because the usual signs and symptoms run a close parallel to potassium intoxication. The latter situation, incidentally, epitomizes the strange ways of electrolyte disturbances; that is, even though the *total* amount of potassium decreases there is an

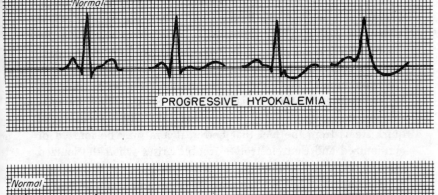

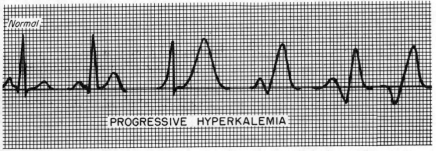

Figure 13: Idealized electrocardiographic tracings showing the effects of hypo- and hyperkalemia.

excess of it in the *extracellular* compartment. Potassium, then, is somewhat like a lion: In its cage, (in the cell) potassium causes no harm, but once out it bites the tissues—severely. The reported symptoms incident to hyperkalemia include listlessness, mental confusion, numbness and tingling of the extremities (with a sense of weakness and heaviness of the legs), a cold gray pallor, hypotension, and characteristic changes in the electrocardiogram.

Calcium

About 99 percent of body calcium is in the bones and teeth, with the remainder in the fluid compartments. A calcium deficit (hypocalcemia) may come about in a number of ways: inadequate intake, poor absorption, hypoparathyroidism, acute pancreatitis, generalized peritonitis, fulminating infection of the subcutaneous tissue, burns and fistulae, to name the more common. What is more, "hypocalcemia" may exist even though the total calcium concentration may be unchanged. This physiological quirk stems from the fact that body calcium may be ionized or non-ionized and that electrolyte trouble arises when the ionized form is converted to the non-ionized form incident to alkalosis. In other words, when we say that the normal calcium content of the extracellular compartment is 4-5 mEq./L., we mean Ca^{++}. This is dramatically underscored in hyperventilation. When excess CO_2 is exhaled the concentration of H_2CO_3 drops and the pH is thereby elevated (respiratory alkalosis). Now, since an increased pH favors the conversion of ionized calcium to the non-ionized variety, the result amounts to a state of hypocalcemia. The classic clinical picture of hypocalcemia is tetany, characterized mainly by muscular twitchings, laryngospasm and generalized convulsions.

Increased concentrations of ionized calcium (hypercalcemia) result from a decrease in pH (either metabolic or respiratory acidosis), renal damage or excessive administration of calcium parenterally. The symptoms are referable to both smooth and skeletal muscles and include constipation, anorexia, dryness of nose and throat, and difficulty in swallowing.

Magnesium

Present in all cells and body fluids, magnesium is involved in calcium and phosphorus metabolism and appears to be closely related physiologically to sodium in that the excretion of both ions seems to be similarly controlled. Magnesium is known to play a vital role in carbohydrate and protein metabolism. Interestingly, there is a definite correlation between the severity of diabetes and the magnesium content of the blood. A deficit of magnesium (hypomagnesemia) leads to cutaneous vasodilatation, twitching of muscles, hyperexcitability, tetany and convulsions. An excess of the ion (hypermagnesemia) can occur when magnesium compounds are administered in the presence of renal failure. The cardinal symptoms include circulatory collapse and respiratory depression.

Phosphate

Because phosphate ($HPO_4^=$) is an important and integral ion of the intracellular compartment and closely allied to calcium, potassium and magnesium, many now believe that the ion should be present in solutions used to replace lost fluids. Further, in the "repair" of hypokalemia of long standing, dipotassium phosphate (K_2HPO_4) would appear to be the electrolyte of choice.

Diagnosis

The physician has three methods at his disposal for estimating the status of body fluids and making a diagnosis of an imbalance in fluid, electrolyte or pH: the patient's history, physical examination and laboratory determinations.

History

The highlights of the history should include estimation of the fluid intake since the onset of disease; estimation of fluid loss since the onset of disease; number of times voiding has occurred in the last twenty-four hours; and, above all, as accurate as possible a recording of weight loss. In the infant and child a loss of 10 percent or less of body weight is considered a moderate fluid deficit, whereas anything above 10 percent ranks as a serious deficit; in larger children and adults moderate and severe deficits result from a loss of 5 percent and over, respectively.

Physical examination

A significant fluid and electrolyte imbalance in most cases will be reflected in the basic signs. In addition to such obvious criteria as alertness, tissue turgor, and the condition of the membranes, the tongue, and the eyes, the physician notes body temperature, respiration, pulse and blood pressure. In dehydration, for example, the picture is one of lethargy, dry membranes, sunken eyes, soft eyeballs, low blood pressure, fast, weak pulse and hypotension. Further, if an acidosis or alkalosis were superimposed upon this disturbance, respiration would be, in most instances, affected—increased or decreased, respectively. For the more subtle alterations in water, electrolytes, and pH the physical examination yields few clear-cut signs and symptoms, but this is not to say that the astute diagnostician will not come away with a lead or two.

Laboratory determinations

The findings in the laboratory are very helpful but must always be considered in the framework of the clinical picture. This is especially true in the case of potassium imbalances, because in the wake of mass tissue destruction the extracellular compartment may actually be hyperkalemic in the face of an overall deficit of that ion. (As pointed out previously, injured cells release intracellular potassium.) Put another way, a blood sample does not always reflect the true state of affairs.

In addition to potassium content, other blood characteristics of importance in establishing a diagnosis include sodium, chloride, carbon dioxide combining power (i.e., HCO_3^-), plasma pH, red cell count, hemoglobin and hematocrit. For example, the classic blood picture incident to severe diarrhea would be one of hyponatremia, hypokalemia, acidosis (low bicarbonate) and an elevated hematocrit (because of hemoconcentration). A urine analysis also reveals considerable information. The pH and acetone will signal an acid-base imbalance; the specific gravity runs high with a fluid deficit; and sugar, albumin, pus and the like, afford clues as to the underlying disease.

VI

THERAPEUTIC PRINCIPLES

Once a given fluid or electrolyte disturbance has been identified, the physician selects the appropriate drug, electrolyte or solution to re-establish balance. If the trouble is edema, diuretics are used to effect the removal of the excess fluid; if a severe acidosis is present, an alkalinizing solution is given; if a severe alkalosis is present, an acidifying solution is given; and so on. Understandably, the bulk of fluid and electrolyte therapy concerns the replacement of lost water and ions, and it is to this area that we shall now direct our attention.

Therapeutic aims

Fluids and electrolytes are given for one, two or all three of the following quite obvious reasons:

1. To replace or "repair" previous losses
2. To provide daily maintenance requirements
3. To replace concurrent losses

Daily maintenance refers to the normal losses via the skin, lungs and kidneys; previous losses refer to those which occurred prior to treatment; and concurrent losses are those which occur during treatment (from vomiting, diarrhea, drainage and gastrointestinal suction).

Nutrition

There is, of course, one point which up until now has not been mentioned, and this is the patient's nutritional requirements over and above water and electrolytes. For minor situations, particularly those where the oral route is available, the intravenous feeding is essentially one of water and electrolytes. However, when the oral route is not available, nitrogen balance and caloric balance take on a therapeutic importance second only to fluid and ions.

Most authorities consider the bedridden patient to have a basal metabolic rate of about one half the normal value and a daily caloric requirement somewhere around 1600 calories. Intravenous solutions are now available which supply these calories (generally as carbohydrates), nitrogen (as amino acids) and those vitamins essential to the metabolism of amino acids and carbohydrates. Also, solutions are available containing ethyl alcohol as an added source of calories. For example, one popular commercial preparation, containing amino acids, invert sugar, and alcohol, supplies approximately 800 calories per liter— a complete meal, with a cocktail, to boot!

The situation in intravenous therapy is epitomized by the man in the desert. His immediate problem is to replace lost water and electrolytes. Next he worries about food.

Dosage

The *volume* of parenteral fluid to be administered in any given imbalance is predicated upon the aims set forth above and the body surface area which is ascertained by the use of the nomograms. (See Part III, numbers 7 and 8.) To satisfy the daily maintenance requirements and repair past losses, three dosages have been established:

Maintenance. 1500 ml. per square meter (M^2) of body surface per day

Maintenance plus moderate previous losses. 2400 ml./M^2/day

Maintenance plus severe previous losses. 3000 ml./M^2/day

These dosage volumes refer to so-called maintenance, or "balanced," solutions, that is, solutions which provide water and electrolyte in amounts which the body can safely handle, assuming normal functioning of the kidneys, adrenals, pituitary and parathyroids. In other words, the body or, more precisely, the kidneys (under the influence of these glands) will retain from such solutions what is needed and reject what is not needed.

Concurrent losses

It is, as indicated, not always sufficient to replace fluid previously lost and to provide daily maintenance needs. If fluids are still being lost, additional replacement is indicated. Such concurrent losses are replaced on a *volume-for-volume* basis, which obviously means that a close check must be made on all fluids the patient loses in an abnormal manner. These should be measured or, if this is not feasible, estimated. Concurrent losses are repaired with special solutions whose composition approximates the electrolyte profile of gastric and intestinal juices. Being more concentrated, these solutions should not be used for previous losses or maintenance therapy.

Routes of administration

Though the subject of fluid and electrolytes brings to mind the gadgetry of intravenous therapy, the simple truth is that whenever practicable the oral route is preferred. Unfortunately, the typical situation requires the parenteral route, and the hazards involved therewith, not to mention the fuss and bother.

Intravenous route

The intravenous route (venoclysis) is the parenteral route of choice and in most instances presents no special problems—in competent hands, of course—provided the patient's cardiovascular and renal systems are functioning normally. Or, put another way, the choice of solution and the rate of administration via this route hinge upon circulatory competence and urine output. In infants and small children the scalp veins are usually most feasible, especially in obese infants in whom it is difficult to insert the needle in veins on the back of the hand (the second site of choice in this age group). In older children and adults the antecubital veins are usually most accessible but there are, as shown in Fig. 14, a number of other excellent sites.

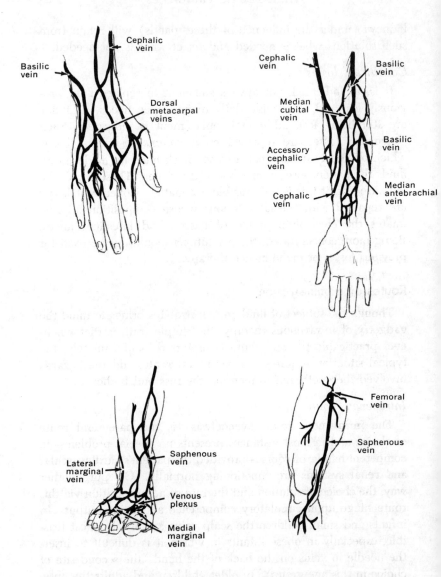

Figure 14: Commonly used and recommended sites for venipuncture. (From *Parenteral Solutions Handbook*, 1965. Courtesy Cutter Laboratories, Berkeley. California.)

Subcutaneous route

For all intents and purposes the subcutaneous route (hypodermoclysis) is the last resort for a number of reasons. The volume of fluid which can be infused is limited; absorption is poor and irregular; and it is uncomfortable to the patient. Moreover, solutions should be isotonic (or very nearly so), low in pH, lightly buffered, and contain no more potassium than the extracellular compartment. Nonetheless, when the administration of parenteral fluids is a matter of life and death and a suitable vein is not available, these obstacles become somewhat academic.

Rates of administration

The rate at which a solution is infused into the bloodstream is of paramount importance. Too fast a rate causes circulatory overload and cardiac failure ("speed shock"), especially in the patient with pre-existing circulatory difficulties. The result can be death. The rates given below are intended merely to be general guides and obviously are subject to individual adaptation.

Initial hydrating solution

Prior to the giving of balanced solutions—or any other solution containing potassium—the kidneys must have demonstrated their ability to excrete urine, and for this purpose hydrating solutions ("low electrolyte, no potassium") are used. However, if urine flow is already established such solutions are not needed. Hydrating solutions are administered at a rate of 8 ml. per square meter per minute (8 ml./M^2/min.) for 45 minutes. If by the end of this time the patient has not voided, the rate is lowered to 2 ml./M^2/min. and continued for another hour. Failure to void at this time may be considered indicative of renal impairment.

Balanced solutions

For maintenance therapy the rate is 2 ml./M^2/min. if given over twenty-four hours or 4 ml./M^2/min. if given in two infusions. (The twenty-four-hour dosage is divided in half and the second half given after a twelve hour interval.) In the correction of previous losses and maintenance the rate is 3 ml./M^2/min.

Gastrointestinal replacement solutions

These solutions, used solely on a volume to volume basis in the replacement, or repair, of concurrent losses, are administered at a rate of 3 ml./M^2/min.

Note: *The rates given above are given in milliliters because of the variation in the different infusion sets. Never assume that the directions for one infusion set apply to any other set!*

VII

SOLUTIONS

All parenteral solutions must be sterile, non-pyrogenic and free from any foreign matter that might cause undesirable reactions. Commercially prepared solutions meet these stringent demands and, almost without exception, are the ones used in our hospitals. The majority are marketed in 500 ml. and 1000 ml. vacuum sealed bottles equipped with a metal bale for suspending the unit. Other sizes include 150 ml. and 250 ml. bottles, and vial concentrates (e.g., Incert and Ion-o-trate). The latter should *never* be used undiluted.

Parenteral solutions are administered by gravity-flow continuous-drop infusion; the rate is ascertained in the sight, or drip, chamber. The complete venoclysis unit contains (in addition to the drip chamber and sterile bottle of solution) rubber or plastic tubing, a safety clamp to regulate flow rate, a needle adapter and needle. Such units are either re-usable or expendable. The re-usable type demands the fuss and bother of cleaning and sterilization—in this day and age a decided hindrance; the expendable type conserves space, time and manpower and affords a simple, standardized method of administration with added safety.

The number and variety of parenteral solutions available is vast and somewhat confusing to the uninitiated unless considered in the framework of a practical bedside system of classification. Moreover, and this is worth remembering, a good 80 percent of parenteral therapy entails nothing more than the old standbys: normal saline, glucose, and glucose in saline. The multiplicity of solutions, therefore, stems from those 20 percent or so special occasions which call for solutions of a more sophisticated content.

47

Carbohydrate–water solutions

This category includes solutions of dextrose (glucose), levulose (fructose) and invert sugar (dextrose and levulose) in plain water, generally in 5 and 10 percent concentrations. By far the most commonly used of these is 5 percent dextrose, the standard parenteral solution for treating dehydration occasioned by a loss solely of water. That is, the dextrose is metabolized leaving plain water to be distributed throughout the various compartments. Obviously, correcting water deficits with electrolyte solutions would incite an electrolyte imbalance by supplying needless ions.

Saline solutions

The solutions in this category include normal saline, "hydrating" solutions and hypertonic solutions. Normal saline, or isotonic sodium chloride solution, is a 0.9 percent solution of that salt and supplies 154 mEq. of sodium and 154 mEq. of chloride per liter. Until recent years normal saline was one of the most widely used electrolyte solutions in parenteral therapy, but now it is often replaced by solutions that physiologically are more beneficial. This is understandable, for whereas the sodium content comes close to that of serum (142 mEq./L.) the chloride content overshoots the mark (103 mEq./L.). Normal saline is most useful in imbalances wrought by gastric suction (with loss of HCl), vomiting due to pyloric obstruction, and excessive sweating.

The so-called hydrating solutions contain sodium chloride in concentrations below that of normal saline; probably the most widely used is 0.45 percent sodium chloride in 2.5 percent dextrose. Such solutions are used, as explained earlier, to initiate therapy in dehydration; that is, they are administered until renal function is adequate, at which time there is a switch over to balanced solutions.

Hypertonic saline solutions contain 3 percent or 5 percent sodium chloride and are employed in those situations where the body has lost more salt than water (i.e., hyponatremia accompanied, usually, by hypochloremia). Too, the 3 percent solution is indicated in the drastic dilution of the plasma following an excessive intake of water. While receiving these potent solutions the patient must be under constant observation. These solutions are contraindicated in the presence of normal, elevated or slightly decreased plasma electrolyte.

Ringer's solution

Ringer's solution contains sodium, potassium, calcium and chloride in amounts approximating those in the extracellular compartment. The solution is indicated following drastically diminished water intake and following increased excretion of water and electrolytes in vomiting, diarrhea, fistula, drainage, and the like. The dose is based on age, weight and clinical condition of the patient.

Lactated Ringer's solution

This preparation (also called Hartmann's solution) approximates the ionic pattern of the extracellular compartment even more than plain Ringer's solution because of its content of lactate. The solution continues to enjoy wide use in meeting fluid deficits and in correcting the compartmental shifts caused by burns, fractures, infection and cardiovascular emergencies. The dose depends upon the age, weight and condition of the patient.

Maintenance solutions

The advent of so-called maintenance, or balanced, solutions has done much to advance fluid and electrolyte therapy by providing a simple, straightforward means of supplying water and electrolytes in just the right amount; that is, 1500 ml. of balanced solution per square meter of body surface will meet the daily requirements of a normal, healthy person for water, sodium and potassium; and, in most instances, 2400 ml./M^2 and 3000 ml./M^2 satisfy the needs in moderate dehydration and severe dehydration, respectively. Butler's solution, or Electrolyte No. 2, the "original" balanced solution, has the following ionic composition:

$$Na^+....55 \text{ mEq./L.}$$
$$K^+....23 \text{ mEq./L.}$$
$$Mg^{++}.... 5 \text{ mEq./L.}$$
$$Cl^-....45 \text{ mEq./L.}$$
$$HCO_3^-....26 \text{ mEq./L.}$$
$$HPO_4^{=}....12 \text{ mEq./L.}$$

Note that although the Na^+ and Cl^- content are low compared to saline and Ringer's solution, the potassium is high, meaning that adequate urinary flow must be established prior to administration. Among the other commonly used balanced solutions are "Electrolyte 75" (for older children and adults) and "Electrolyte 48" (for infants).

Although, as indicated, balanced solutions are useful in most situations—perhaps 80 to 90 percent of all patients—requiring fluid therapy, there are imbalances that cannot be adequately or safely treated in this fashion. These include renal impairment, adrenal insufficiency, hypoparathyroidism, diabetes insipidus, severe exhaustion, severe hypocalcemia, severe acidosis or alkalosis, and severe burns. In these conditions more specific measures are indicated—saline in heat exhaustion, calcium in hypocalcemia, and so on.

Gastrointestinal replacement solutions

Under "Principles of Treatment" we discussed the volume-for-volume replacement of concurrent gastrointestinal losses and their repair through the use of the appropriate replacement solutions. The commonly used solutions of this character are Electrolyte No. 1 (intestinal losses), Electrolyte No. 3 (Cooke and Crowley's Gastric solution), and Darrow's solution (infantile diarrhea). Because these solutions are tailored for specific replacement purposes they should not be used as general purpose balanced solutions. This is especially important to keep in mind in light of the fact that some replacement solutions are sub-labeled "balanced solution." No confusion will ever arise, however, *once the directions are read.*

Alkalinizing solutions

For the correction of metabolic acidosis, 1/6 molar (M/6) sodium lactate solution has been the standard remedy in initial emergency therapy; the dose depends upon the severity of the condition and the patient's weight and age. Because the rationale for this solution depends upon the metabolism of lactate to bicarbonate—in the liver—the solution is contraindicated in liver disease. Other contraindications include alkalosis, shock, and congestive heart failure.

Another agent employed in the treatment of metabolic acidosis is sodium bicarbonate, which is indicated for the rapid correction of the condition, especially in patients with impaired lactate metabolism. The usual preparation is the M/6 solution (1.4 percent $NaHCO_3$). A 7.5 percent solution is used in severe cases when water intake is restricted and also in the emergency treatment of an electrolyte imbalance characterized by hyponatremia and hyperkalemia. Because of the ease with which such solutions overshoot the pH mark, great care must be exercised to avoid alkalosis. In cases where sodium bicarbonate does not produce the desired results, an agent called tromethamine (THAM) is used. The usual preparation is a 0.3 molar (0.3M) solution.

Ammonium chloride

A solution of 2.14 percent ammonium chloride in water is the standard remedy to correct severe states of alkalosis arising from gastrointestinal losses and certain respiratory disturbances, such as emphysema. The mechanism of action is that NH_4^+ is metabolized in the liver to urea and H^+ ions. Throughout the infusion period the patient must be kept under constant watch and a "CO_2 combining power" test must be made of the patient's serum before each infusion. Because it is so easy to cause acidosis with this solution, the rate of administration should not exceed 400 ml. per hour. Ammonium chloride is contraindicated in patients with renal or hepatic failure.

Nutrient solutions

When oral feeding is impractical, caloric and nitrogen balance must be effected through parenteral alimentation, an area of therapy where tremendous strides have been made. For this purpose all sorts of solutions are now available containing amino acids, sugars, alcohol, and vitamins, alone or in combination. Also, balanced electrolyte solutions are invariably charged with sugar. Butler's, or Electrolyte Solution No. 2, for instance, is marketed with 10 percent invert sugar (Fig. 15).

Carbohydrate

Solutions of 5 percent and 10 percent dextrose in water are employed to supply calories and water without electrolytes. For special purposes (e.g., tubular necrosis with oliguria) more concentrated (e.g., 20%) solutions are used. Dextrose solutions with sodium chloride and/or other salts provide electrolyte as well as water and calories. Since 1 gram of monohydrate glucose (the form used in making solutions) supplies 3.4 calories, 1 liter of the 5 percent solution supplies 170 calories, and the 10 percent solution 340 calories. For the adult the 5 percent solution is given at an average infusion rate of 1 liter in 1¼ hours, and the 10 percent solution 1 liter in 3 hours.

Levulose, or fructose, is an isomer of dextrose with the same caloric value. (However, because the anhydrous instead of the hydrous form is used in manufacture, levulose solutions supply a few more calories per liter.) The metabolism of levulose is less dependent upon insulin and less disturbed by stressful situations; thus levulose has an advantage in the presence of fever, diabetes, and liver disease, and following surgery. Furthermore, levulose may be given at double the rate for dextrose; for example, a liter of 10 percent levulose may be given in the same time (1½ hours) as a liter of 5 percent dextrose, and in half the time required for 10 percent dextrose.

Invert sugar (half dextrose and half levulose), in the opinion of some, offers advantages in some cases because it steps up the metabolism of dextrose and thereby enhances overall carbohydrate utilization. Invert sugar solutions are marketed in 5 and

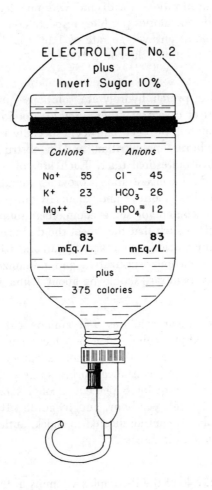

Figure 15: An "all-purpose" solution useful in perhaps 80 to 90 percent of all adult patients requiring fluid therapy. Similar solutions include Electrolyte No. 48 (for the newborn) and Electrolyte No. 75 (for adult therapy).

10 percent concentrations (with and without electrolytes) and supply 190 and 380 calories per liter, respectively. The 5 percent solution is given at an average rate of 1 liter in 1¼ hours, and the 10 percent solution 1 liter in 2 hours.

Amino acids

Amino acid, or protein hydrolysate, solutions (prepared by the acid hydrolysis of casein or other suitable protein) are used to restore and maintain nitrogen balance, especially in wound healing, infection, burns, malnutrition, and in obstruction and diseases of the gastrointestinal tract. Each liter of 5 percent solution (the standard concentration) provides about 40 grams of protein (about 160 calories) and about 18 mEq. of potassium. The electrolyte content of some commercial solutions (for example, Amigen) is such that they meet the daily requirement for electrolyte. Amino acids are marketed plain and with sugar and/ or alcohol. To maximize utilization and minimize nausea and vomiting the average rate should be about 1 liter in 3 hours.

Alcohol

As indicated, sugar solutions and amino acid solutions are available with ethyl alcohol (at a 5 percent concentration) to bolster the caloric intake. Too, alcohol's sedative and analgesic properties are of some assistance during surgery and in obstetrics. The average rate for 5 percent alcohol solutions in children is 50 to 150 ml. per hour, and in adults, 100 to 300 ml. per hour. Alcohol is contraindicated in shock, anticipated shock, epilepsy or severe liver disease.

Vitamins

The essential role of the B-complex vitamins in the metabolism of amino acids, fats and carbohydrate is an established fact. Further, the B-complex vitamins are reported to assist in wound healing and recovery from hemorrhagic shock. Vitamins for parenteral purposes are marketed as concentrates (in ampules) or in standard infusions of normal saline, 5 percent dextrose, and the like.

Blood volume expanders

Controlling shock and acute blood loss is often a matter of life and death. Whole blood is the preferred fluid, but often it is in short supply. There are certain risks involved—transfusion reactions, hyperkalemia (when blood is stored for two to three weeks) and serum hepatitis. Plasma is the next best blood volume expander, especially in the treatment of burns, and has the added feature that there is no need for typing or cross-matching. Closely allied to plasma is human serum albumin or similar plasma fractions (e.g., Plasmanate), which are used occasionally in the treatment of shock, hypoproteinemia, and edema arising from a lack of albumin.

The most commonly used synthetic expander is dextran 75 (a polymer of glucose) which is marketed at a 6 percent concentration in either normal saline or glucose. Aside from its pronounced osmotic properties the advantages of this agent relate to low cost, stability and ease of storage (no refrigeration required). For the adult in shock the usual dose ranges somewhere between 500 and 1000 ml.; in children 250 ml. may suffice. The recommended rate is 20 to 40 ml. per minute.

Dextran 75 at a 12 percent concentration is used to treat edema of nephrosis. In this capacity it acts as an osmotic diuretic.

Dextran 40 (Rheomacrodex), or low molecular weight dextran, is a more recent preparation used for the prevention or inhibition of intravascular aggregation of red blood cells, or the so-called sludging of blood. It appears to increase the suspension stability of blood, which is accompanied by a breaking-up of sludge aggregates, decreased stasis in affected areas, and increased capillary blood flow.

In patients with allergies the dextrans must be used with caution. Nausea, vomiting, wheezing and hypotension have all been reported.

Dialyzing solutions

Although we hear much about the efficiency of the artificial kidney, it is interesting to note that peritoneal dialysis has proved

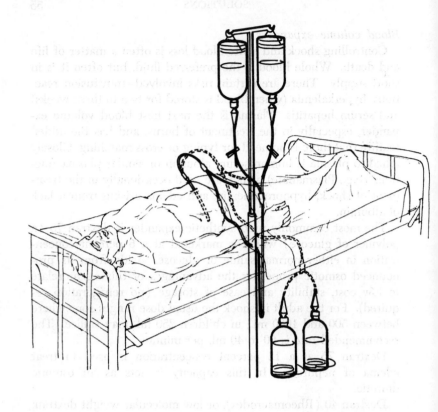

Figure 16: Peritoneal dialysis. Dialyzing solution is infused into abdominal cavity with bottles suspended from stand and drained away with empty bottles placed on the floor. A full course treatment usually requires from 20 to 25 exchanges (i.e., 40 to 50 liters of solution) and takes from 12 to 36 hours. (From *Parenteral Solutions Handbook*, 1965. Courtesy of Cutter Laboratories, Berkeley, California.)

itself useful in areas far removed from the sophisticated gadgetry of the medical center. The technique is safe, inexpensive, exquisitely simple and reasonably efficient. Successful results now have been obtained in renal failure, hyperkalemia, hypercalcemia, excess hydration, and barbiturate and salicylate poisoning.

In peritoneal dialysis the peritoneum serves as the dialyzing membrane; that is, when solutions of the proper composition are introduced into the abdominal cavity (via a closed drainage-paracentesis technique) diffusible wastes, electrolytes, poisons and the like pass from the blood into the solution. The "spent" solution is thereupon withdrawn and replaced with fresh solution (Fig. 16). From this mechanism of action we can readily appreciate the composition of such solutions. They are similar to extracellular fluid except in regard to the absence of potassium and the presence of dextrose; that is, potassium and other wastes diffuse into the solution to establish balance on both sides of the peritoneum, and dextrose renders the solution of sufficient osmolarity to prevent the absorption (of the solution) into the blood. The glucose concentration used depends upon the patient's state of hydration. Cutter Laboratories' Peridial solutions, for instance, are available as Peridial 1½-D (1½ percent dextrose), Peridial 2½-D (2½ percent dextrose) and Peridial 7-D (7 percent dextrose). The "1½-D" is used for patients without edema, and the "2½-D" and "7-D" for patients with moderate and severe edema, respectively.

PART TWO

THE FACTS APPLIED

VIII

AT THE BEDSIDE

Now that we are equipped with the basic facts, let us go to the bedside and treat the patient. Naturally, no two clinical situations are exactly alike; the various measures and procedures presented are merely guidelines to be altered as the physician sees fit.

The surgical patient

In a very real sense the surgical patient is an excellent example to study because his needs dovetail neatly with all that we have said. For instance, let us suppose a male patient with pyloric obstruction enters the hospital in a state of moderate dehydration incident to vomiting, and, further, during the first twenty-four hours incurs a concurrent loss of one liter of fluid via gastric suction. The management of this case, then, entails repair of the previous and concurrent losses plus meeting the daily maintenance requirements of water, electrolyte and calories. Assuming a height of 5′ 8″ and a weight of 140 pounds, the following steps will effect balance for the first twenty-four hours:

1. Using the nomogram (Part III, number 8) we find that the patient has a surface area of 1.75 square meters (M^2) and therefore—based on the physician's assessment of moderate dehydration—needs 1.75 x 2400 ml. or 4200 ml. of solution to cover the previous loss and meet the daily requirement. (Moderate dehydration calls for 2400 ml./M^2/24 hours.)
2. Fluid therapy is initiated with a hydrating solution until renal function is adequate, at which time a balanced solution is started.

61

3. The volume of balanced solution to be given is equal to the estimate made in Step 1 minus the volume of hydrating solution used. For example, if 400 ml. of hydrating solution were given, the volume of balanced solution required would be 3800 ml.

4. The volume of fluid lost via gastric suction is carefully measured and, as indicated, amounts to 1 liter. This volume is repaid by administering 1 liter of replacement solution.

5. The patient's caloric needs for the first twenty-four hours are easily attended to by selecting a balanced electrolyte solution containing sugar. For example, if the 3800 ml. is given as a solution containing 10 percent invert sugar, the patient will receive (counting the sugar in the hydrating solution) about 1500 calories. As compared to many situations one encounters in parenteral alimentation, this caloric intake is more than adequate.

Heat exhaustion

Losses of sodium chloride and water through excessive sweating in nonacclimatized persons results in a serious and sometimes fatal metabolic state referred to as heat exhaustion; the cardinal symptoms include mental confusion, headache, threatened syncope, dizziness, incoordination, lassitude and lethargy. Often cramps of the muscles of the legs or abdomen occur. The temperature may be subnormal or elevated; the pulse is rapid; and the blood pressure may drop—precipitously so on standing. Characteristically, the skin is usually cool and there is profuse sweating—just the opposite of the picture presented in "heat stroke."

If the patient has been drinking water to relieve his thirst the deficit is plainly one of sodium chloride (the so-called "low-salt syndrome"); if the patient has not had access to water the deficit involves water as well as salt. The management of mild cases merely entails rest in a comfortable temperature and the oral administration of mildly salted drinks. In severe cases with collapse, parenteral therapy is usually indicated: hypertonic (5 percent) saline to correct a salt deficit (when the patient has been drinking water) and isotonic saline to correct a deficit of both salt and water. The dosage of isotonic solution is determined as follows:

1. Subtract the patient's serum sodium level (mEq./L.) from the normal value of 142.
2. Estimate extracellular fluid volume (in liters) by taking 15% of body weight in the adult, and 25% of body weight in the infant.
3. Multiply Step 1 value by the Step 2 value (to get the total sodium deficit).
4. Multiply Step 3 value by 1000 and divide by 154 (normal saline has a concentration of 154 mEq./L.) to obtain ml. of normal saline needed. Or:

$$\frac{\text{total sodium deficit x 1000}}{154} = \text{ml. normal saline}$$

For example, to compute the volume of normal saline to restore balance in a 70 kg. patient with a sodium concentration of 122 mEq./L.,

(1). $142 - 122 = 20$ mEq./L. deficit
(2). $0.15 \times 70 = 10.5$ liters (fluid volume)
(3). $20 \times 10.5 = 210$ mEq. (total deficit)
(4). $\dfrac{210 \times 1000}{154} = 1300$ ml. (in round figures)

Burns

A severe burn is as challenging as a severe hemorrhage. Whereas one is prone to think first of destroyed areas, it should not be forgotten that the burn victim is threatened by shock, hypotension, dehydration, electrolyte imbalance and renal impairment. From many textbook descriptions one may ascribe these ominous signs to a loss of fluid. Although there is a loss from the body proper, the amount lost this way is small compared to the fluid which accumulates in and around the burned area; that is, water leaves the circulation through the damaged capillaries and floods the immediate intercellular compartment.

As a result of the water loss from the plasma compartment, there is a drop in blood pressure (due to the drop in blood volume) and hemoconcentration. The drop in pressure contributes to the shock and inhibits the formation of urine, and the hemoconcentration brings about a generalized dehydration by withdrawing intercellular water from the tissues at large. This, of course, happens because a concentrated blood has a greater osmotic pressure. In other words, the fluid of the edematous site is maintained at the expense of the entire body. Since the extent of the edema and actual loss of fluid from the surface depend upon the area and depth of the burn, we can easily appreciate why a burn involving over half the body's surface commonly has a poor prognosis.

The loss of fluid into the damaged tissue proceeds rapidly for the first eight hours following the burn. From then on the flow slows considerably but continues to inundate the site up to about the second day. During the recovery period the displaced water is reabsorbed into the circulation, and the reabsorbed water plus the added volumes of therapeutic fluid causes a copious output of urine somewhere around the third to the fifth day. Consequently, no further fluids should be given until the excesses have been washed away.

A current practice in the restoration of fluid and electrolyte balance in burn patients entails the use of Lactated Ringer's solution, glucose, dextran, plasma, and blood at a dosage derived through "fluid calculators" or tables (Part III, numbers 10 and 11). Looking at these tables note that more blood is needed in third degree burns than in second degree burns, and that dextran may be used in place of plasma. Also, if blood is not available, dextran or plasma may be used on a stopgap basis. The totals (in the tables) cover a twenty-four-hour period and are to be administered as follows: One-half the total volume is given in the first eight hours, one-fourth in the second, and one-fourth in the third eight hour period. (For burns covering an area greater than 50 percent, the dosage is the same as for 50 percent burns.) On the second day, as a rule, the dosage of blood, plasma, dextran and Lactated Ringer's solution is reduced to half. Dextrose remains the same.

Example

Let us assume that a 130 lb. adult has second degree burns of the front of the trunk, half of one leg, and one hand. The therapeutic steps are as follows:

1. Using the "Rule of Nines" (Fig. 17) compute the area:

Front of trunk	18%
Half of leg	9%
Hand	2%
Total area	29%

2. Consult the table: Taking the burned area to be 30% we note under "body weight" of 130 lbs. ("second degree" table):

Lactated Ringer's solution	3600
Dextrose 5%	2500
Toal fluid requirement	6100 ml.

3. Above total fluid requirement to be given as follows during first twenty-four hours:

First 8 hours:	3050 ml.
Second 8 hours:	1525 ml.
Third 8 hours:	1525 ml.

   (Fluids to be given at such a rate as to insure a urinary output of 18-50 ml. per hour)

4. Second twenty-four-hour period:

Lactated Ringer's solution	½ (3600) or 1800 ml.
Dextrose 5%	2500 ml.
Total	4300 ml.

Shock

Shock is perhaps the most baffling medical emergency. Moreover, the ominous signs (hypotension, pallor, clammy skin, feeble pulse, decreased respiration, anxiety, and often unconsciousness)

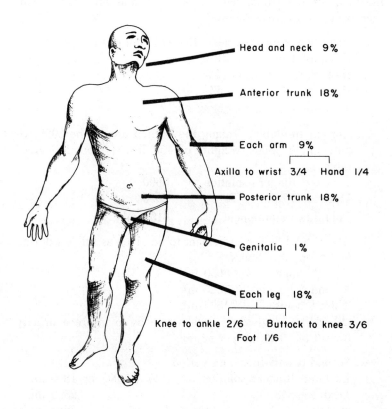

Figure 17: Estimating the burned area (patients 10 years and older) according to the "Rule of Nines." (Redrawn from *Fluid and Electrolytes,* 1960. Courtesy of Abbott Laboratories, North Chicago, Illinois.)

are frightening even to the seasoned physician. Morbidly interesting is the fact that shock is triggered not by one situation, but by many. A severe blow, a burn, a hemorrhage, a heart attack, an unpleasant experience, or even a bee sting may result in shock and death.

From the clinical picture just cited, it is obvious that shock involves the circulation. Moreover, most forms of shock can be explained, at least in part, on the basis of circulatory dynamics. In a severe hemorrhage or burn, for example, the reduced blood volume leads to a reduced venous return and cardiac output. A severe heart attack also causes a drastic cut in cardiaic output because the pump is damaged. In mild shock the body does a reasonable job of protecting itself by constricting the vessels and venous reservoirs. Thus, even though blood may be lost, the constricted vessels maintain normal venous return and cardiac output. If more than a quart of blood is lost, however, this mechanism cannot cope with the task, and cardiac output starts to fall.

The treatment of shock, to be successful, demands speed and proper choice of restorative measures. To correct a volume deficiency, whole blood, plasma, or a plasma expander (for example, dextran) is used. If none of these is available, normal saline solution or 5 percent glucose may be employed. Digitalis is indicated if the heart has been weakened. Although vasocontrictors, such as levarterenol (Levophed) and metaraminol (Aramine), are commonly used to elevate a fallen blood pressure, many authorities nowadays believe that they are of little avail.

The output of urine in shock is much curtailed (because of the drop in blood pressure) and must be corrected before balanced solutions can be given to meet the daily needs of water and electrolyte. Thus, in addition to whole blood, plasma or dextran, one of which is generally given in the initial treatment, hydrating solutions may be required to effect a urine output of at least 20 ml. per hour. For the first twenty-four-hour period, therefore, the volume of balanced solution to be given for maintenance purposes is equal to the calculated volume (e.g., 1500 ml./M^2) minus the total volume of all fluids already administered.

Diabetic acidosis

When for one reason or other the body does not have sufficient insulin to meet its needs, the result is diabetic acidosis, a derangement marked by dehydration, hyponatremia, hypotension, poor renal function, and an acid-base imbalance. In brief, what happens is this: Sugar piles up in the blood (hyperglycemia) and eventually spills over into the urine, taking with it water, sodium and potassium. At the same time the tissues, unable to properly metabolize glucose, start to burn fat at such a rate that acid metabolites ("ketone bodies") accumulate in the blood and decrease the bicarbonate reserve. The kidneys, which ordinarily excrete acids as ammonium salts (to conserve sodium) now are so over-taxed that sodium is lost, thereby aggravating an already existing hyponatremia occasioned by the glucose-induced diuresis. The loss of water leads to a diminished blood volume (hypovolemia) and low blood pressure—and consequently poor renal function. This not only worsens the pH picture because of the failure to excrete acid products but also adds to a paradoxical but nonetheless dangerous hyperkalemia. (It is paradoxical because potassium is *lost* from the cells to the extracellular compartment as a result of faulty metabolism.) Finally, water and electrolyte loss is enhanced by a diminished oral intake of fluid and by vomiting, the latter induced by the ketosis.

The basic treatment of diabetic acidosis entails the administration of insulin and alkali to correct the underlying problem and acidosis, and of hydrating and balanced solutions to repair the deficit of water and electrolyte. Since most clinicians have their own favorite approach to the use of these materials at the bedside, the following represents but one version:

1. Administer an initial dose of regular (unmodified, crystalline) insulin at a dose of 2 units per kilogram of body weight.
2. Administer a hydrating solution (e.g., glucose 5% in sodium chloride 0.45%) plus sodium lactate (50 to 100 mEq./L.) to initiate flow of urine and combat acidosis.

3. Administer (for the remainder of the 24-hour period) a balanced solution at a dose equal to the calculated volume (2400 ml./M² for moderate dehydration and 3000 ml./M² for severe dehydration) minus the volume of solution used in Step 2.
4. Administer whole blood or plasma if necessary.
5. Administer additional insulin on a basis of blood glucose levels.
6. Start fluid (balanced solution plus sugar) by mouth as soon as it can be tolerated.

Edema

Edema means the presence of abnormally large amounts of fluid in the interstitial compartment. The condition is disfiguring, painful, and, not infrequently, a threat to life. A good understanding of the underlying causes is essential to the proper nursing and medical management of the water-logged patient. As indicated, there is no single cause of edema. Indeed, there are few diseases with a greater number of etiologic possibilities. Theoretically, any defect which favors the formation or inhibits the removal of intercellular fluid may be the culprit.

Fluid enters and leaves the intercellular spaces through the capillary wall. Also, a certain amount of tissue fluid is drained away via the lymphatics. (The physical factors which determine the direction of the flow across the capillary were depicted in Fig. 4.) In brief, at the arteriolar end of the capillary the hydrostatic pressure (i.e., blood pressure) normally is greater than the osmotic pressure of the serum protein; consequently, fluid is forced out of the capillary. At the venular end, the hydrostatic pressure drops below the osmotic pressure; consequently, tissue fluid enters the capillary.

Etiology

The defect leading to edema which can be visualized most easily, perhaps, is injured capillary walls, through which fluid *and* protein pour freely into the intercellular compartment. This is an especially troublesome form of edema because the loss of protein not only robs the blood of its power to hold fluid in circulation, but also increases the power of the tissue fluid to take it away. Capillary damage resulting in edema is seen in inflammation and burns, and allergies. Although the edema is usually localized to the area affected, such things as a generalized urticaria or sunburn may cause widespread involvement.

Again, if for any reason the hydrostatic pressure should be elevated at the capillary's venular end, edema will ensue because the return of tissue fluid in the circulation is inhibited. A variety of factors can bring about an elevated venular hydrostatic pressure. Let us start with something as simple as merely *standing*. In this position, the venular pressure in the lower extremities shoots way above the protein osmotic pressure with the result that the legs start to swell. Luckily, this does not happen when moving about because the contraction of the muscles "milks along" the blood through the veins and lymphatics, thereby preventing congestion and an increased venular pressure.

The edema associated with varicose veins occurs whether a person moves about or not because the massaging action of the muscles is of no avail in the face of damaged valves in the vein. Muscle massage is also ineffectual in obstruction of the veins (e.g., thrombophlebitis) and in obesity. In the latter state the fat surrounding the veins insulates the walls from the muscular movement. Probably one of the most common causes of edema in the legs is tight garters. Cutting off the return of venous blood raises the venular pressure even when the body is in full movement.

One of the most serious forms of edema attends the failing heart. Although there is considerable dispute as to the precise mechanism involved, undoubtedly an increased venular pressure is part of the picture. As far as *cor pulmonale* (pulmonary edema of cardiac origin) is concerned, an elevated venous pressure represents the chief etiologic factor. In this condition only the left side of the heart is weak. This means that while the lungs are receiving blood at a normal rate, the blood is not leaving at a normal rate because of the failing left ventricle. The result is congestion, an elevated venous pressure, and a dangerous edema.

Again, a decrease in concentration of plasma protein lowers the osmotic pressure within the capillary to the point where the formation of tissue fluid greatly exceeds its reabsorption into the circulation. Generally speaking, edema occurs when the serum-protein level falls below 5 Gm. per 100 ml. A number of pathologic avenues lead to hypoproteinemia. The more common causes include nephrosis, amyloid kidneys, hepatitis, dehydration, and malnutrition.

If for some reason the lymphatics are obstructed, the flow of lymph is impeded and edema ensues. This is eminently illustrated in elephantiasis, in which filarial worms work their way into the lymphatics and produce almost complete blockage. Other common clinical modes of obstruction include trauma and obesity.

Once edema has started, the condition is soon aggravated and intensified through the influence of aldosterone and the antidiuretic hormone, ADH. Briefly, the sequence of events is as follows: as a result of the loss of fluid to the intercellular compartment, there is a drop in blood volume which in turn stimulates the release of aldosterone and ADH. The former hormone acts on the renal tubule to conserve salt, and the latter to conserve water. This would be physiologically sensible if it were not for the fact that the water and salt so retained are soon lost to the intercellular spaces.

And finally, the kidney also plays a role in edema. As a result of the hypovolemia, (the loss of fluid from the circulation) there is a decrease in renal blood flow and poor filtration. This leads to a retention of salt and an aggravation of the existing condition.

Treatment

To effect the immediate removal of edematous water, diuretics are used—often with life-saving results—to step up the output of urine. And in the instance of those diuretics which have a profound effect upon the elimination of sodium chloride—the so-called "saluretics"—there is also a concomitant drop in blood pressure, especially when they are used in combination with other antihypertensive agents. In addition, saluretics cause an appreciable increase in the output of potassium, which means one must be on the lookout for hypokalemia.

For the emergency treatment of edema, however, the mercurial diuretics are the drugs of choice. A single injection has been known to flush out 10 liters of fluid in twenty-four hours! Four conmmonly used "mercurials" are meralluride (Mercuhydrin), mercaptomerin (Thiomerin), mercurophylline (Mercuzanthin) and chloromerodin (Neohydrin). Once edema is under control through the use of mercurial diuretics the current trend is to switch to the oral saluretics for maintenance therapy if the situation is of a chronic nature. One of the first and still most widely used saluretics is hydrochlorothiazide (marketed as Hydro-Diuril, Enduron, Esidrix, Oretic, and others).

In edema associated with kidney failure diuretics are obviously of no avail, and in this connection hypertonic dialyzing solutions (e.g., Peridial 7-D) may be life-saving.

Water intoxication

While one could hardly be criticized for referring to edema as "water intoxication," the latter designation is reserved for those situations where water accumulates *within* the cell; that is, whereas edema is an *extracellular* accumulation of fluid, water intoxication is an *intracellular* accumulation.

When greater amounts of water are taken into the body than the kidney and obligatory losses can balance, the extracellular compartment swells, causing a lowering of osmotic pressure. As a result, water leaves the intercellular spaces and invades the cells. Essentially, this is the same pathological picture as seen in the low-salt syndrome, and many of the signs and symptoms are identical. The principal repercussions include confusion, drowsiness, muscle twitching and coma. Characteristically, the skin is moist, warm and flushed. Generally, there is no edema.

Since few people care enough about water to imbibe to the point of intoxication, we might well wonder where this situation is encountered. Interestingly, most cases occur right in the hospital. It will be recalled that the stress of trauma, surgery, anesthesia and the like stimulates the release of ADH, resulting in the retention of water, and, if during this period there is an excess intake of water without salt (e.g., forced fluids) a state of intoxication will result.

Treatment

Once the condition has been identified, the administration of fluids should be stopped immediately, and, as an aid in mobilizing the trapped water, small amounts of concentrated salt solutions given. This procedure stimulates diuresis and, therefore, the removal of water.

Polyuria

The passage of abnormally large amounts of urine is direct evidence of the kidney's inability to conserve water. Polyuria leads to a generalized dehydration and sometimes acidosis. The chief renal derangements so characterized are chronic nephritis and diabetes insipidus.

Chronic nephritis

In this condition the kidneys put out a highly dilute urine because they have lost their power to concentrate the solute. There is a marked tendency toward dehydration and a degree of acidosis. The replacement of existing water losses is the most important therapeutic measure. For example, if a patient has a urine output of 2.5 L. and 1 L. of normal evaporation loss, 3.5 L. of fluid will be required to maintain balance throughout a twenty-four-hour period.

The daily intake of protein should not exceed the point needed to maintain balance. At 0.6 Gm. per Kg. of body weight, this amounts to about 40 Gm. To minimize protein catabolism—thereby keeping urea and other waste products at a low level—the patient should receive at least 100 Gm. of glucose. This precaution is based upon the biochemical fact that the body, in deriving its energy, prefers glucose over protein; that is, glucose "spares" protein. In general, therefore, chronic nephritis calls for a diet rich in carbohydrate and fat and poor in protein. Fat also "spares" protein.

Another valuable measure in chronic nephritis is the reduction of phosphate. As phosphate is one of the principle anions excreted by the kidney, removing it will lighten the load on that organ. Since milk furnishes large amounts of the ion, it is best left out of the diet or stringently restricted. (If the patient is given supplemental vitamins, minerals and calcium, the omission of milk will not prove of consequence.) A further step in this direction is the administration of aluminum hydroxide (e.g., Amphojel), which sequesters intestinal phosphate and prevents absorption into the circulation.

Provided there is no edema or other complication, salt need not be restricted. Indeed, in the face of a hyponatremia, hypertonic saline is indicated. In general, the wisest approach is to make the best possible appraisal of the body's salt loss and adjust the intake.

Diabetes insipidus

In this derangement the body may lose as much as 15 L. of water per day. As explained previously, the etiologic factor is a lack of the antidiuretic hormone (ADH) from the posterior pituitary. ADH stimulates the renal tubules to reabsorb water, thereby reducing the output of urine and conserving water. It is easy to understand that a deficiency of the hormone tends to dry up the extracellular compartment. As a consequence of the prodigious loss of water, there results great thirst, voracious appetite, loss of strength and emaciation. Indeed, the drinking of 10 to 15 liters of water is debilitating in itself.

It is to be noted that diabetes insipidus has nothing to do with diabetes mellitus. The two diseases share the name "diabetes" because both are characterized by polyuria. The Greek word "diabetes" means *siphon,* and that it is. The term "mellitus" pertains to honey; "insipidus"—meaning tasteless or flat—indicates that the urine in this condition is without sugar.

The treatment of diabetes insipidus is not only successful but also highly dramatic. By giving the appropriate dose of ADH, also called vasopressin (Pitressin), the pathologic flood is brought to a sudden halt. The drug is administered intramuscularly in a dose of 0.3 to 1 ml. every 36 to 48 hours. Treatment must be continued indefinitely to keep the patient asymptomatic.

IX

THE INFANT

The younger we are, the wetter we are. The human embryo is composed of 97 percent water—about the same as a cucumber! The newborn averages about 75 per cent water, compared to the 60 percent figure of adulthood. But since this "excess fluid" of infancy is almost entirely contained in the extracellular compartment, it is rapidly lost from the body via insensible perspiration. Indeed, the week-old baby is already well along on life's road of more or less progressive dehydration.

Physiological considerations

Relative to the adult, the infant has a greater water need and greater water loss and adjusts much less promptly to alterations in fluid and electrolyte. In round figures, whereas the adult has a water turnover of about 45 ml. per kilogram per day the three-month-old baby puts out and takes in 150 ml. per kilogram per day (Fig. 18). (For example, using these figures, a 7 kg. infant has an intake and loss of 150 x 7 or 1050 ml. per day, and a 70 kg. adult 45 x 70 or 3150 ml. per day.) Consequently, dehydration, occasioned by disease, and overhydration, occasioned by excessive intake and administration of fluids and solutions, are much more critical and serious in the infant. In the main, the infant's plight in these cases stems from a proportionately greater surface area, higher metabolism, and immature renal performance.

Assuming a 70 kg. adult has a surface area of 1.73 square meters and a 7 kg. infant has a surface area of 0.38 square meter, we can see that the ratio of weight to surface in the adult is 40 to 1 in contrast to a ratio of 18 to 1 in the infant. Thus, proportionately the infant has a surface area between 2 and 3 times (40÷18)

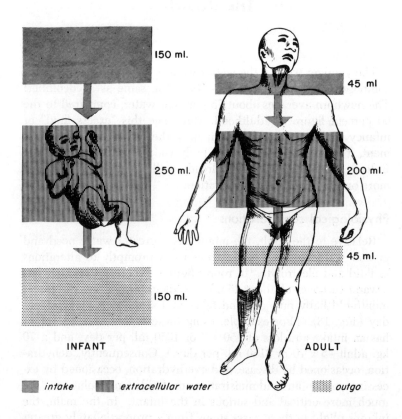

150 ml.

45 ml

250 ml.

200 ml.

45 ml.

150 ml.

INFANT

ADULT

▓ intake ▓ extracellular water ▒ outgo

Figure 18: A comparison of approximate daily water exchange (per kilogram of body weight) in infant and adult. (Redrawn from *Fluid and Electrolytes*, 1960. Courtesy of Abbott Laboratories, North Chicago, Illinois.)

that of the adult and therefore a much greater loss of water through the skin. And since the metabolic rate and heat production are allied to surface area, the infant also outdoes the adult in this regard—with a rate two to three times greater per kilogram of body weight. This means, of course, a relatively greater production of metabolic wastes and hence proportionately greater output of urine. The urine output in the infant is also enhanced by the inefficiency of the immature kidney. Indeed, the immature kidney is relatively unable to either conserve or excrete water easily after excessive intake. Another renal defect relates to acid-base balance; that is, hydrogen ions are much less easily excreted (as NH_4^+) than in the adult. As a result, the infant can easily pass into acidosis unless the diet is carefully watched. Diets yielding high fixed-acid residues are to be especially avoided.

Sodium and potassium go hand in hand with the rapid exchange of water. For instance, in periods of fever and starvation the sodium content is easily reduced to dangerous levels. Conversely, in diarrhea, where more water is lost than salt, the resulting hypernatremia is poorly managed by the immature kidney. As a matter of fact, the immature kidney fails to cope with any sudden rise in electrolyte.

Therapeutic points

From the above, then, we can well appreciate that the management of fluid and electrolyte balance in the pediatric patient affords much less room for error than in the adult. It is an easy matter to give too little or too much. However, the principles of therapy for children and adults are the same; our purpose here is to consider certain additional points.

Diarrhea

Because of the speed with which fluid and electrolyte are lost from the intestinal tract—resulting in circulatory collapse and impaired renal function—diarrhea in the infant will always constitute a serious problem. Definitive treatment depends upon the degree of dehydration and type of dehydration. In the vast majority of diarrheas the result is isotonic dehydration—meaning equivalent losses of water and electrolyte. Hypertonic dehydration, on the other hand, arises from a proportionately greater loss of water than electrolyte. Here the child shows irritability rather than lethargy (characteristic of the isotonic variety) and may go into convulsions. In hypotonic dehydration, the least common type, the loss relates more to electrolyte than water, and the condition is materially worsened by taking plain water. The situation here, paradoxically, has overtones of water intoxication because the drop in osmotic pressure in the extracellular compartment causes water to pass into cells, producing overhydration in that compartment.

Mild cases of diarrhea very seldom necessitate the use of parenteral solutions provided due attention is given to the oral route. Milk and other feedings are withheld at the outset and, in their place, well tolerated liquids are given to supply water and electrolyte. For example, 5 percent dextrose in half strength saline or sweetened tea with one-half teaspoonful of salt to a quart of water (at a dose of 200 to 300 ml. per kilogram of body weight) may be given for the first twenty-four hours. After this period, boiled skim milk diluted with equal parts water and sweetened with sugar is alternated with such solutions to afford an intake in the next twenty-four hours of 150 to 120 ml. per kilogram of body weight.

In severe diarrhea with toxic symptoms and circulatory failure a sample of blood is taken for laboratory analysis (CO_2 combining power, pH, sodium, potassium) and administration of an isotonic solution (e.g., Lactated Ringer's solution) started at once and continued over the first hour at a dose of 20 ml. per kilogram. If this does not correct the shock, whole blood at a dose of 10 ml. per kilogram is given over the second hour. As soon as the sodium concentration is known and the nature of dehydration characterized, the following solutions are recommended over the next 6 to 8 hours to repair the deficit:

Isotonic dehydration:

    Darrow's solution (60 ml./kg.) and

    Dextrose 5% (40 ml./kg.)

Hypotonic dehydration:
   Darrow's solution (60 ml./kg.) and
   Dextrose 5% in Lactated Ringer's solution (40 ml./kg.)

Hypertonic dehydration:
   Sodium lactate (M/6) (20 ml./kg.),
   Dextrose 5% (60 ml./kg.) and
   Potassium and calcium (according to laboratory report)

Once the deficit has been repaired a balanced solution is given at a dose of 1500 ml./M^2/24 hours to supply maintenance needs (and is continued until oral feedings are retained), and further concurrent stool losses are corrected using 5 percent dextrose and Darrow's solution.

Pyloric stenosis

Even though surgery is considered the ultimate answer to pyloric stenosis, its success in any given case depends upon the preoperative restoration of fluid and electrolyte balance. And this is a real challenge, for the continued vomiting which characterizes this condition deprives the body of prodigious amounts of chloride (as HCl) and water. Proportionately less sodium and potassium is lost. Moreover, the loss of acid results in an alkalosis which "de-ionizes" serum calcium and, in severe cases, causes tetany. In a compensatory attempt to correct the condition, respiration may be depressed to elevate plasma carbonic acid, but in severe cases this mechanism is inadequate. Thus, the picture is ominous—dehydration, alkalosis, hypochloremia, hyponatremia, hypokalemia and hypocalcemia.

The first order of business is to treat the tetany by giving calcium gluconate at a dose of 0.5 ml. to 1 ml. per kilogram of body weight and the appropriate "acidifying solution" to correct the alkalosis. Brief inhalation of 5 percent carbon dioxide (95 percent oxygen) is also helpful. Hydrating solutions are given next (300 ml./M^2 for the first forty-five minutes of treatment) to initiate the flow of urine and, once this is accomplished, a balanced solution is started. The dose is 3000 ml./M^2/24-hours minus the volume of hydrating solution given. Once the deficit has been repaired and the crisis is over, the balanced solution is given at the regular maintenance dose of 1500 ml./M²/24-hours. If surgery is performed, however, there must be a switch to potassium-free hydrating solutions.

In instances where the obstruction is below the pylorus, or in association with diarrhea, the result may be acidosis rather than alkalosis because of the loss of alkaline secretions. In this instance, M/6 sodium lactate solution is employed to initiate treatment.

Burns

As we might well imagine burns in the infant and child are more severe than in the adult, and those covering an area of 10 percent or more almost always necessitate parenteral therapy. Aside from a special "Rule of Nines" (Fig. 17), however, the basic therapy is the same as in the adult; that is, plasma, dextran, Lactated Ringer's solution, dextrose and blood are administered on a basis of weight, surface area and severity of burn.

Salicylate poisoning

The first symptom in this very common poisoning (aspirin is the usual culprit) is rapid and deep breathing caused by the direct action of the drug on the respiratory center. Other initial effects often seen are extreme thirst, vomiting, profuse sweating, fever, and confusion or delirium. Later, as the state of intoxication becomes more intense, there is circulatory collapse, oliguria (or anuria), hemorrhage, coma and convulsions. Interestingly, the initial respiratory alkalosis—stemming from the hyperventilation—gives way to an acidosis stemming from renal shutdown. The treatment consists of gastric lavage; cold sponging to reduce the fever; vitamin K to arrest bleeding; oxygen to support the brain and kidney; and parenteral solutions to supply sodium, potassium, and water and to stem the falling pH. Incidentally, alkaline solutions (sodium lactate or sodium bicarbonate) augment the elimination of salicylates.

X

ACUTE KIDNEY FAILURE

An extensive survey reported by Lucké in 1946 brought to light that a wide variety of pathological situations terminate in acute renal failure (also referred to as acute renal insufficiency and acute tubular necrosis). It is now generally established that this ominous derangement often follows in the wake of nephrotoxic poisonings, burns, shock, trauma, and transfusion reactions.

The chief sign is a drastic cut in the output of urine (oliguria); sometimes no urine is formed at all (anuria). The reason for this response is not hard to understand. In the case of nephrotoxic poisons (e.g., carbon tetrachloride) the tubular epithelium—principally at the proximal end—undergoes degeneration and desquamation. As a result, the glomerular filtrate, instead of being acted upon by a metabolically selective lining, passively diffuses back into the bloodstream.

Although the same pathologic mechanism prevails in the other forms of renal shutdown cited above, the tubular lesions in these instances are more diffuse, commonly extending all the way along to the collecting tubules. Moreover, some nephrons may be spared while others are totally destroyed. Consequently, oliguria rather than anuria is the rule.

The anuric patient is in delicate balance between life and death. The cause of death is generally an excess of potassium (hyperkalemia), aided and abetted by acidosis and excess fluid (hypervolemia). Before anything can be said concerning the management of this challenging malady, it is essential to briefly discuss these three features.

81

Hyperkalemia

Although one might be prone to think that *urea,* the chief urinary waste product, is the main culprit in acute kidney failure, most evidence points to potassium. Both laboratory and clinical data show that the cardinal signs and symptoms of renal shutdown usually run parallel to those of potassium intoxication.

Potassium is no doubt the most sensitive ion of the extracellular compartment, for only a few milliequivalents either way from the normal value of 4-5 mEq./L. plunge the body into a precarious state. This deviation is the crux of the entire syndrome; the very small amount released from the cell (as a consequence of protein catabolism) is—in the presence of renal failure—great enough to cause poisoning. In other words, even on a potassium-free diet the exodus of the K^+ ions continues to insult the extracellular environment with increasing vigor. Even at a level of only 7 mEq./L. the body is in serious trouble. While certain measures (to be discussed under *Treatment*) are of value in delaying the rise in concentration, all efforts will fail unless there is a return of renal sufficiency.

It cannot be emphasized too strongly that potassium intoxication arises from *extracellular* phenomena; that is, the body may succumb to potassium even though the *total* amount of the ion in the body remains the same. The principal repercussions of renal shutdown—or hyperkalemia—are seen in the nerves, muscle and the heart; these include muscular weakness, paralysis, paresthesias and cardiac impairment. The usual cause of death is cardiac standstill.

Cardiac action

The heart will not function in the absence of potassium. Experimental hearts stop beating—in systole—when perfused with fluid containing all the essential ions except K^+. By adding the correct amount of potassium the embarrassment is readily removed. At the other extreme, too much potassium also stops the heart—but in diastole. From studies such as these, researchers have shown that potassium plays two roles in myocardial physiology: it affects the transmission of impulses and it affects muscle contraction. Provided the extracellular level remains at 4-5 mEq./L., potassium plays these roles to the body's benefit.

The effects of hypokalemia and hyperkalemia, as indicated earlier, are reflected in the EKG (Fig. 13). As long ago as 1938, Winkler and his colleagues showed very clearly that electrocardiographic tracings follow a set pattern in the face of an increasing serum K^+. Although these workers obtained their results by infusing potassium chloride into dogs, the picture in man has proved to be essentially the same. While the EKG is of obvious value in the study of cardiac action in potassium derangements, it should not be taken as the last word in the diagnosis of potassium intoxication. Only the serum potassium levels afford unequivocal results.

Acidosis

Acute anuria leads to acidosis because the disabled kidney is unable to excrete hydrogen ions released in the metabolic processes. As a result the accumulating ions unite with HCO_3^-, producing an excess of carbonic acid (H_2CO_3) and a decrease in the HCO_3^- to H_2CO_3 ratio.

Hypervolemia

Because the anuric individual can lose no more than one liter of water per day via insensible perspiration, the fluid intake must be cut drastically. Otherwise, the circulation swells (hypervolemia) beyond safety and edema ensues. Excess fluid, in the form of pulmonary edema, may well cause death. Since the patient's water loss is met in part (300 to 400 ml.) by the release of water from damaged tissue and oxidation of endogenous fat and protein, the present practice is to keep the fluid intake at about 500 cc. In the event of abnormal skin losses or gastrointestinal losses, additional fluid is administered.

Treatment

The sole idea behind the treatment of the anuric individual is to maintain a state of "normalcy" throughout a precarious period.

In the event the failure is reversible, intelligent therapy will have saved a life. The specific points to watch are the following:

Fluid

Unless there are abnormal losses, the daily allowance should not exceed 500 ml. for the totally anuric patient. Amounts greater than this will produce hypervolemia and possibly pulmonary edema. Fluid is best given intravenously as hypertonic glucose (see the next point—*Diet*).

Diet

The diet should be free of potassium, protein, and, in the absence of extracellular losses, sodium. To minimize the breakdown of tissue protein, the caloric intake must be balanced to meet basal requirements. Failure to do so means disaster, because the release of potassium in protein catabolism will severely aggravate the existing hyperkalemia. And yet, even with these precautions there is an inevitable accumulation of the ion. At best, then, all one can do is to delay the attainment of dangerous K^+ levels. Besides potassium, protein breakdown also releases acidic products. This spells acidosis and contributes to the anuric syndrome.

The caloric requirement is best met by the intravenous administration of 40 percent glucose; to avoid venous thrombosis, the solution should be given by continuous drip through a plastic catheter inserted into a large vein. In a dose of 500 ml., the daily fluid allotment, a 40 percent solution delivers 200 Gm. of glucose, or 680 calories. Authorities agree that at least 100 Gm. of glucose are needed to spare protein, that is, minimize its breakdown.

On the above regimen the body weight ought to decrease about $\frac{1}{4}$ to $\frac{1}{2}$ lb. per day. Whenever the patient maintains his weight, it indicates that too much fluid is being administered. The best guide to successful therapy, therefore, is a daily weighing. This is an important nursing procedure, and to be of value it must be done accurately.

Cation exchange resins

The advent of the so-called cation exchange resins has contributed significantly to the management of renal anuria. The type resin used contains exchangeable sodium ions; that is, when the resin is placed in contact with fluid containing the K^+ ion, the latter is exchanged for Na^+.* This principle had been employed for years in the softening of water before it was put to use at the bedside.

When used properly, these agents are a valuable aid in the management of hyperkalemia. The resin, in the course of its sojourn through the intestinal tract, removes the K^+ ion from the juices therein and ultimately brings down the extracellular potassium. The usual dose is 50 gm. daily. If the oral route cannot be used, the resin may be added to water and given rectally. Of course, the volume of water used must be subtracted from the daily requirement to avoid hypervolemia.

Dialysis

When the above conservative measures fail in any vital area the artificial kidney (hemodialysis) or peritoneal dialysis must be considered, the latter being much less efficient than the former, but having a decided advantage when heparinization is contraindicated. In addition, peritoneal dialysis is inexpensive, uncomplicated and always available; in areas far removed from a medical center it may be the one last hope.

The major types of artificial kidney in clinical use today include the "twin-coil," the "stationary sheet," the "parallel flow" and the "rotating drum" (Fig. 19). All, of course, operate on the principle of dialysis, that is, small molecules ("crystalloids") pass through cellophane but large molecules ("colloids") do not. Referring to Figure 19, we see that as the blood courses through the cellophane tubing the cells and protein remain within but the waste products diffuse into the bath, the latter charged with electrolytes—but not potassium—and glucose at concentrations approximating those of the blood. Thus, the blood is cleaned but not devitalized.

---

* The resins employed to remove sodium in edema contain exchangeable hydrogen and potassium.

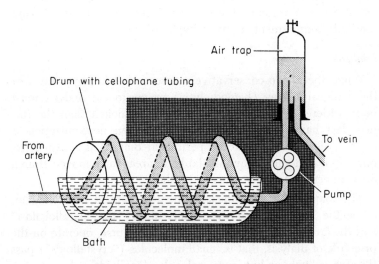

Figure 19: After Maclean, from Brooks, S. M. *Integrated Basic Science*, 2nd edition. C. V. Mosby, Co., 1966.

Prognosis

Blood urea nitrogen (BUN) concentrations offer reliable estimates of the kidney's progress toward recovery because they pretty much reflect the overall renal performance. A drop in BUN, accompanied by reasonable volumes of urine, offers a favorable prognosis. Sometimes the kidneys may excrete a urine little modified by the renal tubules so that vital constituents of the glomerular filtrate are lost because of the poor absorption, signifying that management of the immediate post-anuric phase demands close attention to the loss of water, protein and electrolyte.

REFERENCES

Anderson, J. A. Fluid therapy in infants and children. *J. Lancet*, 1947, *67*, 185.

Baskin, J. L., Keith, H. M., and Scribner, B. H. Water metabolism in water intoxication—Review of basic concepts. *Am. J. Dis. Child.*, 1953, *83*, 618-627.

Belinkoff, S., and Hall, O. W. Alcohol solutions. *Am. J. Obst. Gynec.*, 1950, *59*, 429.

Black, D. A. K. Body-fluid depletion. *Lancet*, 1953, *1*, 353.

Bland, J. H. *Clinical Recognition & Management of Disturbances of Body Fluids*, 3rd Ed. Philadelphia: W. B. Saunders Co., 1962.

Blocker, T. G., Levin, W. C., Nowinski, W. W., Lewis, S. R., and Blocker, V. Nutrition studies in the severely burned. *Ann. Surg.*, 1957, *141*, 589.

Brooks, S. M. The ABC's of water and electrolyte balance. *J. Nurs. Ed.*, 1962, *1*, 13.

Brooks, S. M. *Basic Facts of Pharmacology*, 2nd Ed. Philadelphia: W. B. Saunders Co., 1963.

Brooks, S. M. *Integrated Basic Science*, 2nd Ed. St. Louis: C. V. Mosby Co., 1966.

Brooks, S. M. *Basic Facts of General Chemistry*. Philadelphia: W. B. Saunders Co., 1956.

Bull, J. P., and England, N. W. J. Fluid and electrolyte exchange in patients with burns. *Lancet*, 1954, *2*, 9-17.

Burns, R. O., Henderson, L. W., Hager, E. B., and Merrill, J. P. Peritoneal dialysis. *N. Eng. J. Med.*, 1962, *267*, 1060-1066

Butler, A. M. Parenteral fluid therapy in diabetic coma. *Acta Paediat.*, 1949, *38*, 59.

Chatton, M. J., Margen, S., and Brainserd, H. *Handbook of Medical Treatment*. Los Altos: Lange Medical Publications, 1964.

Clinical applications of fluid and electrolyte balance. *Physicians Bulletin*. Indianapolis: Eli Lilly Co., 1961.

Cooke, R. E., and Crowley, L. G. Gastrointestinal replacement solutions. *N. Eng. J. Med.*, 1952, *246*, 637.

Danowski, T. S. Fundamental features of metabolism of sodium and potassium. *Am. J. Clin. Path.*, 1953, *23*, 1095.

Danowski, T. S., et al. Studies in diabetic acidosis and coma, with particular emphasis on the retention of administered potassium. *J. Clin. Invest.*, 1949, *28*, 1.

Darrow, D. C. Body-fluid physiology: the role of potassium in clinical disturbances of body water and electrolyte. *N. Eng. J. Med.*, 1950, *242*, 978.

Darrow, D. C., Pratt, E. L., Fleet, J., Gamble, A. H., and Wiese, H. F. Disturbances of water and electrolyte in infantile diarrhea. *Pediatrics*, 1949, *3*, 129.

Darrow, D. C., and Pratt, E. L. Fluid therapy, relation to tissue composition and the expenditure of water and electrolyte. *J.A.M.A.*, 1950, *143*, 365.

DeSanctis, A. G., and Varga, C. *Handbook of Pediatric Medical Emergencies*, 2nd Ed. St. Louis: C. V. Mosby Co., 1956.

Editorial. *J.A.M.A.*, March 26, 1949, *139*, 850.

Elkinton, J. R., and Danowski, T. S. *The Body Fluids*. Baltimore: The Williams and Wilkins Co., 1955.

Ellison, E. H., Morgan, T. W., and Zollinger, R. M. Practical aspects of potassium therapy in the surgical patient. *Ohio Med. J.*, 1951, *47*, 839.

Elman, R. Postoperative complications due to electrolyte disturbances. *Postgrad. Med.*, 1952, *11*, 202.

Elman, R. *Surgical Care*. New York: Appleton-Century-Crofts, Inc., 1951.

Elman, R., et al. Intracellular and extracellular potassium deficits in surgical patients. *Ann. Surg.*, 1952, *136*, 111.

Fluid and electrolytes. North Chicago: Abbott Laboratories, 1960.

Fluid therapy. Morton Grove, Ill.: Baxter Laboratories, Inc., 1962.

Fratkin, L. B. Potassium deficiency in surgical patients. Paper read before the British Columbia Surgical Society, Vancouver, B.C., March 31, 1951.

Gamble, J. L. *Chemical Anatomy, Physiology, and Pathology of Extracellular Fluid*. Cambridge: Harvard University Press, 1950.

Gaspar, M. R. The potassium problem in surgery. *Am. Surg.*, 1952, *18*, 524.

Geyer, R. P. Parenteral nutrition. *Physiolog. Rev.*, 1960, *40*, 150.

Gillespie, C. E. Potassium deficiency and hypochloremic alkalosis in the postoperative patient. *Am. Surg.*, 1952, *18*, 1109.

Goodman, L. S., and Gilman, A. *The Pharmacological Basis of Therapeutics*, 2nd Ed. New York: Macmillan, 1958.

Hoffman, W. S. Clinical physiology of potassium. *J.A.M.A.*, 1950, *144*, 1157.

Holliday, M. A., and Segar, W. E. The maintenance need for water in parenteral fluid therapy. *Pediatrics*, 1957, *19*, 823.

Ivy, A. C., Greengard, H., Stein, I. F., Jr., Grodins, F. S., and Dutton, D. G. Effect of various blood substitutes in resuscitation after otherwise fatal hemorrhage. *Surg., Gynec., and Obst.*, 1943, *76*, 85-90.

Kane, F. C. Sodium imbalance. (Staff conference at Salem, Mass., Hospital, December, 1949.)

Knowles, H. C., Jr., and Kaplan, S. A. Treatment of hyperkalemia in acute renal failure using exchange resins. *A.M.A. Arch. Int. Med.*, 1953, *92*, 189-194.

Lans, H. S., Stein, I. F., Jr., and Meyer, K. A. Diagnosis, treatment and prophylaxis of potassium deficiency in surgical patients. *Surg. Gyn. Obst.*, 1952, *95*, 321.

Marriot, H. L. *Water and Salt Depletion.* Springfield: Charles C Thomas, 1950.

Maxwell, M. H. and Kleeman, C. R. *Clinical Disorders of Fluid and Electrolyte Metabolism.* New York: McGraw-Hill, 1962.

Mayer, C. A. *Fluid Balance, A Clinical Manual.* Chicago: Year Book Publishers, 1952.

Mayer, J. H. Diuretics. *Seminar Report* (Merck Sharp and Dohme Research Laboratories), Spring 1958, 2-9.

Merrill, J. P. *The Treatment of Renal Failure.* New York: Grune and Stratton, 1955.

Miller, D. G. A guide to parenteral fluid therapy. *Mil. Surg.*, 1952, *111*, 253.

Moyer, C. A. *Fluid Balance.* Chicago: Year Book Publishers, 1952.

Nelson, W. E. *Textbook of Pediatrics,* 7th Ed. Philadelphia: Saunders, 1959.

Newburgh, L. H. *Significance of the Body Fluids in Clinical Medicine.* Springfield: Charles C Thomas, 1950.

New and nonofficial remedies, report of Council on Pharmacy and Chemistry. *J.A.M.A.*, 1954, *154*, 241.

Overman, R. R. Sodium, potassium, and chloride alterations in disease. *Physiol. Rev.*, 1951, *31*, 285.

Parenteral Solutions Handbook. Berkeley, Calif.: Cutter Laboratories, 1965.

Patton, R., Ellison, E. H., Boles, E. T., and Zollinger, R. M. Potassium depletion in surgical patients. *Arch. Surg.*, 1952, *64*, 726.

Peters, J. P. Diabetic acidosis. *Metabolism.* 1952, *245*, 847.

Peters, J. P. Regulation of the volume and composition of body fluids. *J. Missouri M. A.*, 1950, *47*, 9.

Peters, J. P. Water balance in health and disease. In Duncan, G. G. *Diseases of Metabolism,* 2nd Ed. Philadelphia: Saunders, 1947.

Schwartz, W. B., Levine, H. D., and Relman, A. S. Electrocardiogram in potassium depletion. *Am. J. Med.*, 1954, *16*, 395.

Schwartz, W. B., and Relman, A. S. Acidosis in renal disease. *N. Eng. J. Med.*, 1957, *256*, 1184.

Scribner, B. H., and Burnell, J. M. *Syllabus for the Course on Fluid and Electrolyte Balance.* Seattle: University of Washington School of Medicine, 1960.

Smith, H. W. *Principles of Renal Physiology.* New York: Oxford University Press, 1956.

Snively, W. D., and Sweeney, M. J. *Fluid Balance Handbook for Practitioners.* Springfield: Charles C Thomas, 1956.

Statland, H. A. A fluid and electrolyte balance service for clinical use. *J.A.M.A.,* 1952, *150,* 771.

Statland, H. A. *Fluids and Electrolytes in Practice,* 2nd Ed. Philadelphia: Lippincott, 1957.

Steele, J. M. Body water. *Am. J. Med.,* 1950, *9,* 141.

Strickler, J. H., Rice, C. O., and Treloar, A. E. Observations on the relationship of output to intake for total fluids, nitrogen, potassium, sodium and chloride for perisurgery patients under parenteral nutrition. *Surgery,* 1956, *49,* 152.

Tarail, R., and Elkinton, J. R. Potassium deficiency and the role of the kidney in its production. *J. Clin. Invest.,* 1949, *28,* 99.

Vest, S. A., and Kelly, R. A. Modern treatment of acute renal failure. *J. Urol.,* 1953, *69,* 55-56.

Wallace, A. B. The treatment of burns. *Practitioner,* 1953, *170,* 109.

Water and Electrolyte Metabolism in Relation to Age and Sex. Colloquia on Aging. Vol. 4, Ciba Foundation. Boston: Little, Brown, 1958.

Webster, D. R., Henrikson, H. W., and Currier, D. J. Effect on potassium deficiency on intestinal motility and gastric secretion. *Ann. Surg.,* 1950, *132,* 20.

Weisberg, H. F. *Water, Electrolytes, and Acid-Base Balance.* Baltimore: Williams and Wilkins, 1962.

Wilkinson, A. W. *Body Fluids in Surgery,* 2nd Ed. Baltimore: Williams and Wilkins, 1960.

Wolf, A. V. Body water. *Scientific American,* November, 1958, pp. 125-132.

Wolf, A. V. *Thirst: Physiology of the Urge to Drink and Problems of Water Lack.* Springfield: Charles C Thomas, 1959.

PART THREE

THE FACTS AT A GLANCE

1

THE IONS

Formula	Valence	Atomic or Formula Weight	Equivalent Weight	Milliequivalent Weight
Na^+	1	23	23	0.023
K^+	1	39	39	0.039
Mg^{++}	2	24.3	12.2	0.012
Ca^{++}	2	40	20	0.020
Cl^-	1	35.5	35.5	0.036
HCO_3^-	1	61	30.5	0.031
$HPO_4^=$	2	96	48	0.048
$SO_4^=$	2	96	48	0.048

(handwritten annotations):

$X \text{ equ/li} = \dfrac{W_g}{A/v}$ $\dfrac{W}{100}$? $1 \text{ Eq} = \dfrac{A}{v}$ — atomic weight, per liter — valence

$X \text{ milli equ} = \dfrac{1}{1000} \dfrac{W}{A/v}$ $1 \text{ milli Eq} = \dfrac{A}{1000 V}$ — wt in gr.

$\text{no. milli E} = \dfrac{W \times 1000 \times v}{A}$

2

AVERAGE BODY CONTENT OF WATER AND IONS

| | Adult (70 kg.) | | Child (10 kg.) | |
	Total Content	Daily Exchange	Total Content	Daily Exchange
Water	42 L.	2.5 L.	6 L.	1 L.
Sodium	65 gm.	3 gm.	10 gm.	0.4 gm.
Potassium	175 gm.	3.5 gm.	14 gm.	2 gm.
Chloride	85 gm.	4 gm.	15 gm.	0.5 gm.

3

TYPICAL DAILY WATER EXCHANGE IN ADULT

	Intake		Output
Drink	1650 ml.	Urine	1700 ml.
Preformed water	750 ml.	Skin	500 ml.
Oxidative water	350 ml.	Lung	400 ml.
		Feces	150 ml.
	2750 ml.		2750 ml.

4

AVERAGE ELECTROLYTE COMPOSITION OF GASTROINTESTINAL SECRETIONS AND EXCRETIONS (mEq./L./24 hours)*

	Na^+	K^+	Cl^-
Saliva	9	26	10
Gastric juice (fasting)	60	10	85
Pancreatic fistula	141	5	76
Biliary tract fistula	148	5	101
Intestinal secretion	111	5	104
Ileostomy (recent)	129	11	116
Ileostomy (old)	46	3	21
Cecostomy	79	20	45
Ileum suction	117	5	105
Stools — children			
normal	1	4	0.5
severe diarrhea	12	18	8

*Adapted from Bland, J.H.: *Clinical Recognition and Management of Disturbances of Body Water*, 2nd Ed. Saunders, 1956.

5

AVERAGE PLASMA VALUES FOR ELECTROLYTES

Ion	mg. %*	mEq./Liter†
Na^+	325	140
K^+	20	5
Ca^{++}	10	5
Mg^{++}	2	2.5
Cl^-	360	103
$HCO_3^=$	60 Vol.	27

*i.e., milligrams per 100 ml.

†mEq./L., or milliequivalents per liter are computed from mg.% by the following formula:

$$mEq./L. = \frac{mg.\% \times valence \times 10}{atomic\ weight}$$

For example: Substituting the average normal mg.% for Ca^{++} we have:

$$mEq./L. = \frac{10 \times 2 \times 10}{40} = 5$$

97

6

AVERAGE VALUES FOR NORMAL URINE (24-hour sample)

Volume: 1500 ml.
Transparency: Clear
Odor: "Characteristic" (ammoniacal upon standing)
Specific gravity: 1.015 – 1.020
Acidity: pH 6 (range 4.8 – 7.5)
Total Solids: 60 gm.

Ammonia	0.7 gm.
Calcium	0.2 gm.
Chlorides (as NaCl)	12 gm.
Creatine	0.03 gm.
Creatinine	1.4 gm.
Magnesium	0.1 gm.
Potassium	2 gm.
Sodium	4 gm.
Urea	30 gm.
Other	9.6 gm.

7

NOMOGRAM FOR ESTIMATING SURFACE AREA OF INFANTS AND YOUNG CHILDREN

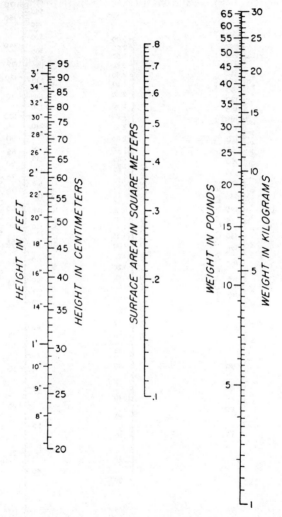

Surface area is found by drawing a straight line between a point representing weight and that representing height. (Reprinted by permission of the publishers from N.B. Talbot, et al., *Functional Endocrinology From Birth Through Adolescence*. Cambridge, Mass.: Harvard University Press, copyright 1952 by the Commonwealth Fund.)

8

NOMOGRAM FOR ESTIMATING SURFACE AREA OF OLDER CHILDREN AND ADULTS

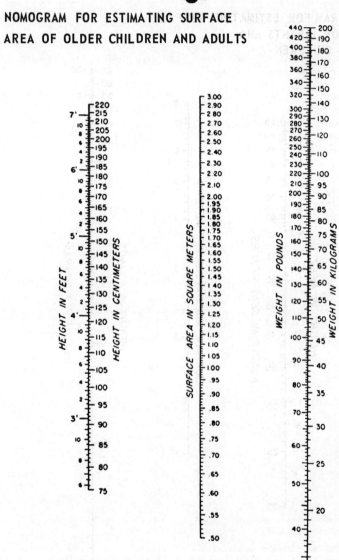

Surface area is found by drawing a straight line between a point representing weight and that representing height. (Reprinted by permission of the publishers from N.B. Talbot, et al., *Functional Endocrinology From Birth Through Adolescence*. Cambridge, Mass.; Harvard University Press, copyright 1952 by the Commonwealth Fund.)

9

AN ALTERNATE METHOD FOR CALCULATING DAILY MAINTENANCE REQUIREMENTS*

Halliday and Segar have proposed an excellent and easily memorized system for maintenance therapy which obviates the use of any type of table or chart. They assume that the average bedfast hospitalized patient has a level of metabolism roughly halfway between the basal state and that of normal activity and, further, that for each Calorie metabolized the body requires 1 milliliter of water, and for each 100 Calories 3 mEq. of sodium, 2 mEq. of potassium and 2 mEq. of chloride. The other point to remember is this:

1) up to 10 kg. (weight) assume 100 Cal./kg.
2) between 10 and 20 kg. assume 1000 Cal./kg. plus 50 Cal. for each kg. over 10 kg.
3) over 20 kg. assume 1500 Cal./kg. plus 20 Calories for every kg. over 20.

Example: What are the daily maintenance requirements of a bedfast 60 kg. adult?
1) the caloric requirement is 1500 + 20 x 40 or 2300 Calories
2) the water requirement is 2300 ml.
3) the electrolyte requirement is as follows:

$$\text{sodium} = \frac{2300}{100} \times 3, \text{ or } 69 \text{ mEq.}$$

$$\text{potassium} = \frac{2300}{100} \times 2, \text{ or } 46 \text{ mEq.}$$

$$\text{chloride} = \frac{2300}{100} \times 2, \text{ or } 46 \text{ mEq.}$$

*From *Clinical Applications of Fluid and Electrolyte Balance.* Physician's Bulletin, Eli Lilly and Company, Indianapolis, 1961.

7okg human being
contains about 3500 mEq of K

10

SECOND DEGREE BURNS: FLUID INTAKE AND OUTPUT*

Body Weight		20	30	40	50	60	70	80	90	100	110
	Kg.	20	30	40	50	60	70	80	90	100	110
	Lb.	45	65	90	110	130	155	175	200	220	240
Recommended Urinary Output, Range in ml.		8-26	11-32	13-38	16-45	18-50	19-56	20-60	22-64	22-66	23-68
Per cent of Skin Burned	Therapy										
20%	Plasma or GENTRAN solution	—	—	—	—	—	—	—	—	—	—
	Lactated Ringer's Solution	800	1200	1600	2000	2400	2800	3200	3600	4000	4400
	Dextrose 5% in Water	1350	1700	1900	2200	2500	2800	3000	3200	3300	3400
	Total	2150	2900	3500	4200	4900	5600	6200	6800	7300	7800
30%	Plasma or GENTRAN solution	—	—	—	—	—	—	—	—	—	—
	Lactated Ringer's Solution	1200	1800	2400	3000	3600	4200	4800	5400	6000	6600
	Dextrose 5% in Water	1350	1700	1900	2200	2500	2800	3000	3200	3300	3400
	Total	2550	3500	4300	5200	6100	7000	7800	8600	9300	10,000
40%	Plasma or GENTRAN solution	200	300	400	500	600	700	800	900	1000	1100
	Lactated Ringer's Solution	1400	2100	2800	3500	4200	4900	5600	6300	7000	7700
	Dextrose 5% in Water	1350	1700	1900	2200	2500	2800	3000	2800	2000	1200
	Total	2950	4100	5100	6200	7300	8400	9400	10,000	10,000	10,000
50% or more	Plasma or GENTRAN solution	500	750	1000	1250	1500	1750	2000	2250	2500	2500
	Lactated Ringer's Solution	1500	2250	3000	3750	4500	5250	6000	6750	7500	7500
	Dextrose 5% in Water	1350	1700	1900	2200	2500	2800	2000	1000	—	—
	Total	3350	4700	5900	7200	8500	9800	10,000	10,000	10,000	10,000

11

THIRD DEGREE BURNS: FLUID INTAKE AND OUTPUT*

Body Weight	Kg.	20	30	40	50	60	70	80	90	100	110
	Lb.	45	65	90	110	130	155	175	200	220	240
Recommended Urinary Output, Range in ml.		8-26	11-32	13-38	16-45	18-50	19-56	20-60	22-64	22-66	23-68
Per cent of Skin Burned	Therapy										
20%	Blood	200	300	400	500	600	700	800	900	1000	1100
	Plasma or GENTRAN solution	200	300	400	500	600	700	800	900	1000	1100
	Lactated Ringer's Solution	400	600	800	1000	1200	1400	1600	1800	2000	2200
	Dextrose 5% in Water	1350	1700	1900	2200	2500	2800	3000	3200	3300	3400
	Total	2150	2900	3500	4200	4900	5600	6200	6800	7300	7800
30%	Blood	300	450	600	750	900	1050	1200	1350	1500	1650
	Plasma or GENTRAN solution	300	450	600	750	900	1050	1200	1350	1500	1650
	Lactated Ringer's Solution	600	900	1200	1500	1800	2100	2400	2700	3000	3300
	Dextrose 5% in Water	1350	1700	1900	2200	2500	2800	3000	3200	3300	3400
	Total	2550	3500	4300	5200	6100	7000	7800	8600	9300	10,000
40%	Blood	400	600	800	1000	1200	1400	1600	1800	2000	2200
	Plasma or GENTRAN solution	400	600	800	1000	1200	1400	1600	1800	2000	2200
	Lactated Ringer's Solution	800	1200	1600	2000	2400	2800	3200	3600	4000	4400
	Dextrose 5% in Water	1350	1700	1900	2200	2500	2800	3000	2800	2000	1200
	Total	2950	4100	5100	6200	7300	8400	9400	10,000	10,000	10,000
50% or more	Blood	500	750	1000	1250	1500	1750	2000	2250	2500	2500
	Plasma or GENTRAN solution	500	750	1000	1250	1500	1750	2000	2250	2500	2500
	Lactated Ringer's Solution	1000	1500	2000	2500	3000	3500	4000	4500	5000	5000
	Dextrose 5% in Water	1350	1700	1900	2200	2500	2800	2000	1000	—	—
	Total	3350	4700	5900	7200	8500	9800	10,000	10,000	10,000	10,000

*From *Fluid Therapy*. Baxter Laboratories, Inc., Morton Grove, Illinois, 1962. Used by permission.

12

SALT AND SUGAR

Solution	mEq./L.	Calories
Sodium chloride 0.45%	Na 77; Cl 77	–
Sodium chloride 0.9% (normal saline)	Na 154; Cl 154	–
Sodium chloride 3%	Na 513; Cl 513	–
Sodium chloride 5%	Na 855; Cl 855	
Dextrose 5%	–	170
Dextrose 2½% and sodium chloride 0.45%	Na 77; Cl 77	85
Dextrose 2½% and normal saline	Na 154; Cl 154	85
Dextrose 5% and sodium chloride 0.45%	Na 77; Cl 77	170
Dextrose 5% and normal saline	Na 154; Cl 154	170
Dextrose 10% and normal saline	Na 154; Cl 154	340
Dextrose 20% and normal saline	Na 154; Cl 154	680
Dextrose 25% and normal saline	Na 154; Cl 154	850
Dextrose 5% and alcohol 5%	–	450
Dextrose 5%, alcohol 5% and normal saline	Na 154; Cl 154	450
Dextrose 5% and potassium chloride 0.2%	K 27; Cl 27	170
Invert sugar 5%	–	187
Invert sugar 10%	–	374
Invert sugar 5% and normal saline	Na 154; Cl 154	187
Invert sugar 10% and normal saline	Na 154; Cl 154	374
Levulose 5%	–	187
Levulose 10%	–	374
Levulose 10% and normal saline	Na 154; Cl 154	374

13
MULTIPLE ELECTROLYTE

Solution	mEq./L.	Calories
Darrow's Solution	Na 122; K 35; Cl 104; HCO_3 54	–
Electrolyte #1 and invert sugar 10%	Na 80; K 36; Ca 4.6; Mg 2.8; Cl 63; HCO_3 60	374
Electrolyte #2 and invert sugar 10% (Butler's Solution)	Na 55; K 23; Mg 5; Cl 45; HCO_3 26; HPO_4 12	374
Electrolyte #3 and invert sugar 10% (Cooke and Crowley's Solution)	Na 63; K 17; NH_4 70; Cl 154	374
Electrolyte #48 and dextrose 5%	Na 25; K 20; Mg 3; Cl 22; HCO_3 23; HPO_4 3	170
and fructose 5%	Na 25; K 20; Mg 3; Cl 22; HCO_3 23; HPO_4 3	187
and fructose 10%	Na 25; K 20; Mg 3; Cl 22; HCO_3 23; HPO_4 3	374
Electrolyte #75 and dextrose 5%	Na 40; K 35; Cl 40; HCO_3 20; HPO_4 15	170
and fructose 5%	Na 40; K 35; Cl 40; HCO_3 20; HPO_4 15	187
Ordway's Solution	Na 26; K 27; Cl 53	123
Potassium chloride 0.3% sodium chloride 0.45% and invert sugar 10%	Na 77; K 40; Cl 117	374
Ringer's Solution	Na 147; K 4; Ca 4.5; Cl 156	
and dextrose 2½%	Na 147; K 4; Ca 4.5; Cl 156	85
and dextrose 5%	Na 147; K 4; Ca 4.5; Cl 156	170
and dextrose 10%	Na 147; K 4; Ca 4.5; Cl 156	340
Lactated Ringer's Solution (Hartmann's Solution)	Na 130; K 4; Ca 3; Cl 109; HCO_3 28	
and dextrose 2½%	Na 130; K 4; Ca 3; Cl 109; HCO_3 28	85
and dextrose 5%	Na 130; K 4; Ca 3; Cl 109; HCO_3 28	170
and dextrose 10%	Na 130; K 4; Ca 3; Cl 109; HCO_3 28	340

14

PROTEIN HYDROLYSATE

Solution	mEq./L.	Calories
Protein hydrolysate 5%	Na 4; K 18	175
Protein hydrolysate 5% and dextrose 5%	Na 4; K 18	345
Protein hydrolysate 5%, alcohol 5% and dextrose 5%	Na 4; K 18	625

15

ACIDIFYING AND ALKALINIZING

Solution	mEq./L.
Ammonium chloride 0.9%	NH₄ 169; Cl 169
Ammonium chloride 2.14%	NH₄ 400; Cl 400
Sodium lactate (M/6)	Na 167; HCO₃ 167*

*Lactate metabolized to HCO_3

16

TONICITY

Solutions which have the same osmotic pressure as the plasma are isotonic. Those with a lower osmotic pressure are said to be hypotonic, and those with a higher osmotic pressure, hypertonic. (Only in isotonic solutions do cells retain their shape.) Tonicity depends upon the number of particles or osmols of solute; that is to say, solutions containing the same number of osmols are isotonic.

One mole (i.e., the molecular weight in grams) of any *nonelectrolyte* in solution is equal to one osmol. On the other hand, the osmolarity of electrolytes depends upon the number of ions formed. Thus, one mole of sodium chloride yields one mole-ion of Na^+ and one mole-ion of Cl^- and therefore a total of 2 osmols. Again, one mole of $CaCl_2$ in solution yields one mole-ion of Ca^{++} and two mole-ions of Cl^- and therefore a total of 3 osmols:

$$CaCl_2 \longrightarrow Ca^{++} \quad + \quad 2Cl^-$$

1 mole   1 mole-ion   2 mole-ions

In physiological and clinical work the osmol is too large a unit so the milliosmol (mOs.) is used. This is equal to 1/1000 of an osmol.

17

REACTIONS WHICH MAY FOLLOW PARENTERAL FLUID ADMINISTRATION*

Cause	Reaction	Clinical Manifestations	Factors Increasing Susceptibility	To Prevent or Minimize Reaction
Elements Contained in the Fluid	Pyrogenic Embolic Vasomotor	Rise in temperature Severe chills Cyanosis Circulatory collapse	Febrile diseases Liver diseases Hypoproteinemia	Use only sterile, pyrogen-free solutions and apparatus
	Post-transfusion hepatitis	Homologous serum jaundice		Use pasteurized blood fractions
Method of Administration	Speed reactions	Circulatory overload Cardiac failure	Cardiac decompensation	Avoid too rapid administration
	Embolic	Air embolism		Replace air in tubing with solution before injecting. Stop injection with 2 or 3 cc. still remaining in receptacle
	Thrombotic	Trauma to walls of vein	Poor nutritive state Low serum protein level	Avoid constant use of same vein
	Tissue necrosis	Edema		Reduce fluid volume Be sure needle remains constant in vein
Specific Incompatibility of Recipient	Hemolytic	Chills Nausea, vomiting Lumbar pain Abdominal cramps Oliguria	Blood group incompatibility Rh type incompatibility Hemolytic anemia	Administer cross-matched blood
	Allergic	Urticaria Angioneurotic edema Asthma	Recipient sensitivity to allergens in donor plasma	Interrupt infusion at first sign of reaction

*From *Parenteral Solutions Handbook*, 1965.
Used by permission of Cutter Laboratories, Berkeley, Calif.

GLOSSARY

acid. A chemical that in solution dissociates into hydrogen ions; a proton donor.

acid-base balance. The biochemical state of the body characterized by a normal pH (7.35-7.4) of the blood.

acidosis. An acidemia or a lowered blood bicarbonate with a tendency toward acidemia.

acute renal failure. A disease of the kidney characterized by either a drastic cut in output of urine (oliguria) or by no urine at all (anuria).

aldosterone. The chief adrenal cortical hormone that stimulates the kidney to conserve sodium and excrete potassium.

alkalinizing solutions. Parenteral solutions used to combat acidosis.

alkalosis. An alkalemia or an increased blood pH with a tendency toward alkalemia.

aluminum hydroxide. A medicinal used to decrease the gastrointestinal absorption of phosphate.

amino acids. Organic acids containing both the amino (NH_2) and carboxyl (COOH) group; the "building blocks" of protein.

anion. A negative ion.

antidiuretic hormone (ADH). A hormone produced by the anterior pituitary that stimulates the kidney to conserve water; also called *vasopressin.*

anuria. The absence of excretion of urine from the body.

artificial kidney. A mechanical device (operating on the principle of dialysis) used to remove wastes from the blood during kidney failure.

balanced solutions. General purpose solutions used in the maintenance of water and electrolyte balance.

109

base. An acceptor of hydrogen ions or protons.

blood urea nitrogen (BUN). A test that indicates the amount of urea in the blood; reflects renal function.

Blood volume expanders. Parenteral solutions used to maintain blood volume in shock.

buffers. Agents—usually consisting of a weak acid and one of its salts—that resist a change in pH.

Butler's solution. A multiple electrolyte solution employed in the treatment of dehydration.

cation. A positive ion.

cation exchange resins. Synthetic resins used to decrease the absorption of potassium from the gastrointestinal tract.

compartment. A theoretical division of the body's water.

Darrow's solution. A multiple electrolyte solution employed to supply lost fluid and potassium in diabetic acidosis and infantile diarrhea.

dehydration. The clinical condition resulting from an undue loss of water.

dextran. A starchy polymer of glucose used as a plasma expander.

diabetes insipidus. A metabolic disorder, marked by great thirst and the passage of a large amount of urine (with no excess sugar) caused by an insufficient output of the antidiuretic hormone.

diabetes mellitus. A metabolic disorder due to a lack of insulin and characterized by hyperglycemia, glycosuria, polydypsia, and polyuria.

dialysis. The process of separating a mixture of crystalloids and colloids via a semipermeable membrane such as cellophane.

diuretics. Drugs used to stimulate the formation of urine.

edema. The abnormal accumulation of fluid in the tissues.

electrolyte. Any substance that furnishes ions in solution. Clinically, a term referring to body anions and cations.

electrolyte balance. The state of the body in relation to the intake and output of electrolytes.

equivalent weight. The atomic weight (in grams) divided by the valence.

extracellular compartment. The fluid of the plasma and interstitial spaces collectively.

gastrointestinal replacement solutions. Special solutions used to replace fluids lost in vomiting and diarrhea.

glomerular filtrate. The aqueous non-protein fluid produced by the glomerulus of the nephron.

glomerulus. The tuft, or coil, of blood capillaries of the nephron.

glucose. A monosaccharide, or simple sugar.

glycosuria. The presence of an abnormal amount of glucose in the urine.

heat exhaustion. A condition caused by excessive heat and marked by subnormal temperature, moist skin, dizziness, nausea, and sometimes, collapse.

hemodialysis. The use of the artificial kidney.

heparinization. The administration of heparin to decrease the blood's ability to coagulate.

homeostasis. The tendency toward stability in the amount and concentration of blood fluids.

hydrating solutions. Low electrolyte solutions used to initiate intravenous therapy in dehydration.

hypercalcemia. An excess of blood calcium.

hyperchloremia. An excess of blood chloride.

hyperglycemia. An excess of blood sugar.

hyperkalemia. An excess of blood potassium.

hypermagnesemia. An excess of of blood magnesium.

hypernatremia. An excess of blood sodium.

hypertonic dehydration. Dehydration in which, proportionately, the loss of water exceeds the loss of electrolyte.

hypertonic solution. A solution of greater osmotic pressure than one with which it is compared.

hypertonic saline. A sodium chloride solution with a concentration greater than 0.9 percent; usually refers to the 3- and 5 percent solution.

hypervolemia. An abnormal increase in blood volume.

hypocalcemia. A decrease in blood calcium.

hypochloremia. A decrease in blood chloride.

hypodermoclysis. The infusion of fluids into the subcutaneous tissues.

hypokalemia. A decrease in blood potassium.

hypomagnesemia. A decrease in blood magnesium.

hyponatremia. A decrease in blood sodium.

hypopotassemia. A decrease in blood potassium.

hypotonic dehydration. Dehydration in which the loss of electroylte proportionately exceeds the loss of water.

hypotonic solution. A solution of lower osmotic pressure than one with which it is compared.

hypovolemia. A decrease in blood volume.

insensible perspiration. Water lost from the lungs and skin via vaporization.

intercellular compartment. The body water or fluid which surrounds the cells.

interstitial fluid. See *intercellular compartment.*

intracellular compartment. The body water within the cells.

ion. An electrically charged atom.

isotonic dehydration. Dehydration characterized by a proportionate loss of water and electrolyte.

isotonic sodium chloride. A 0.9 percent solution of sodium chloride; normal saline.

ketone bodies. Refers to acetone, aceto-acetic acid, and beta-hydroxy-butyric acid (the intermediates in fat metabolism): also called *acetone bodies.*

ketosis. A condition marked by excessive formation of ketone bodies in the body.

kilogram. One thousand grams; 2.2 lbs.

Lactated Ringer's solution. A multiple electrolyte solution commonly used to replace lost fluid.

liter. One thousand milliliters; abbreviated ml.

low-salt syndrome. A condition caused by a drop in the salt concentration of the body's extracellular fluid.

maintenance solutions. Intravenous solutions used to maintain fluid and electrolyte balance.

mercurial diuretics. Potent diuretics containing mercury in organic combination.

milliequivalent. One thousandth of an equivalent; abbreviated mEq.

nephritis. Inflammation of the kidneys.

nephron. The anatomic and physiologic unit of the kidney.

nitrogen balance. The state of the body in relation to the ingestion of nitrogen (as protein) and excretion of nitrogen (as urea, etc.)

nonthreshold substances. Those constituents of the glomerular filtrate not appreciably reabsorbed by the renal tubules.

oliguria. A scanty output of urine in relation to the fluid intake.

osmoreceptors. Receptors of the hypothalamus sensitive to changes in osmotic density.

osmosis. The passage of water through a semipermeable membrane separating two solutions, the chief flow being from the less dense to the more dense.

oxidative water. The water produced in the oxidative metabolism of food.

parenteral. By injection.

parenteral solutions. Sterile solutions used in intravenous therapy.

peritoneal dialysis. The removal of wastes from the blood (during kidney failure) using the peritoneum as the dialyzing membrane.

perspiration. Sweating; the functional excretion of sweat.

pH. A measure of acidity or alkalinity equal to the logarithm of the reciprocal of the hydrogen-ion concentration (per liter of solution). For example, a solution containing 10^{-3} gram-ion of hydrogen per liter has a pH of 3.

plasma compartment. The water of the plasma.

plasma expander. A parenteral fluid used to maintain blood volume in shock.

polyuria. The passage of abnormally large amounts of normal urine.

preformed water. The water present in food.

pyloric stenosis. Hypertropic obstruction of the pyloric orifice of the stomach (usually congenital) resulting in protracted vomiting, dehydration and alkalosis.

Ringer's solution. A solution containing 8.6 Gm. NaCl, 0.3 Gm. KCl and 0.33 Gm. $CaCl_2$ per liter of water.

"Rule of Nines." The area of the body expressed as follows: head, 9 percent (of body area); arm, 9 percent; leg, 18 percent; front of body 18; back, 18 percent.

saluretic. A diuretic that stimulates the elimination of large amounts of sodium.

shock. A condition of acute circulatory failure due to derangement of circulatory control or loss of circulating fluid; brought about by injury.

specific gravity. The weight of a substance divided by the weight of an equal volume of water.

speed shock. The shock-like state resulting from the too rapid administration of parenteral solutions.

sudoriferous glands. Sweat glands.

tetany. A condition marked by muscle twitchings, cramps, and convulsion; caused by hypocalcemia.

INDEX

115